Mental Health Wisdom Book Website:
www.mentalhealthwisdombook.com

Author's Blog: www.antonysimpson.com

This book is for:

All those affected by mental illness. The 25%.

All those who care about someone who has experienced or has a mental illness. The 75%.

Everyone.

Dedicated to all those who have lost their lives due to mental illness.

Dedicated to all those affected by another person's suicide.

Contents

Part 3 - Life Hacks

Forward

I deal with mental health every day. Whether that's my own, someone else's or both. Whether we realise it or not, we all do.

I'm an Alcohol Specialist Nurse by profession. Many of the patients that I see use alcohol to self-medicate the symptoms of an underlying mental illness. The problem with this coping strategy is that self-medication isn't selective. You numb everything, the good as well as the bad. That is without mentioning the other impacts that alcohol has on physical health and their lives. It's like trying to cure a disease by drinking a poison that will ultimately be fatal.

After battling with highs, lows and mixed mood states through my teenage years and early adulthood, I was diagnosed with Cyclothymia (a form of bipolar) at the age of twenty-nine.

In my professional and personal life, I've learned a lot about mental health and illness. This book has been years in the making. I am proud to share my knowledge and experiences with you in this book.

This book is deliberately titled Mental Health *Wisdom* rather than Mental Health *Knowledge*. Wisdom is taking the lessons learned from knowledge and life experiences and applying them in a meaningful way to your life.

There are three parts to this book. In Part 1 - Understanding, I share knowledge I've learned about mental health and illness.

In Part 2 - Empathy Through Lived Experience, I share my

experiences of mental health and illness.

In Part 3 - Life Hacks, I share ways to improve your mental health, as well as ways to prevent and manage mental illness. These life hacks are intentionally short, only giving you the absolutely essential information. Apply these in the way you think will be most helpful in your life.

By gaining knowledge, learning from my experiences and implementing the life hacks you will become mental health *wise*.

Emergency Help

If you are in a mental illness crisis, I ***strongly*** encourage you to access crisis support. A mental illness crisis usually involves:

- Thinking about or planning suicide.
- Self-harm.
- Thinking about or having taken an overdose.
- Feeling completely overwhelmed.
- Severe mood swings.
- Strong and sometimes uncontrollable impulses.
- Hallucinations - visual, audio or tactile.
- Losing touch with reality.
- Psychosis.

In the UK crisis support is available by attending your nearest Accident & Emergency Department. There you can speak to a mental health specialist. They are experts in dealing with mental illnesses and *will* be able to help you.

Remember that thoughts, moods and impulses fluctuate and change. What you think and how you feel now, will not always be how you think and feel.

Part 1 - Understanding

Mechanics of the Mind

I'm fascinated by how the brain functions. That written, I am neither a Neurologist nor a Neuroscientist. Neuroscience as a field of study is in its infancy. However we have identified parts of the brain, how neurons communicate and specific chemicals that make us think, feel and behave in the ways in which we do.

The Parts of the Brain

The brain is split into different parts called lobes:

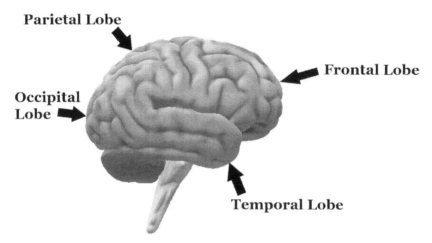

The frontal lobe deals with logical thinking and reasoning. It enables us to develop plans and solve problems. It gives us the ability to predict and imagine outcomes of events before doing them. There's never been a chocolate made that tastes like vomit. Why? Because we can imagine that it wouldn't taste good.

A vital role of this ability to predict and imagine outcomes is empathy. To be able to imagine how others think and feel.

The frontal lobe is also associated with speech, voluntary movement, personality and behaviours linked into the reward pathway. It has the highest numbers of dopamine-sensitive neurons. See more about dopamine and the reward pathway under The Chemical Players section of this chapter.

The parietal lobe deals with interpreting and processing sensory information from our five senses (sight, smell, touch, taste & sound). It also gives us the ability to calculate sums in our head.

The occipital lobe mostly focuses on interpreting and processing visual information. What we see. The colours, light, movement, distance and depth perception. It also helps us to read and understand what we read.

The temporal lobe deals with memory (although the frontal lobe, parietal and occipital lobe all also have a role in the creation, processing and recall of memories), hearing, understanding what we hear, speech, recognising people and emotional responses.

The limbic system is responsible for all of our emotions. It sits mostly in the temporal lobe. It is sometimes called our emotional brain or reptilian brain. It is responsible for the reward pathway, being alert for danger, stress, the Fight, Flight or Freeze Response (see more below), sex, love and caring. All the systems for survival of the individual and survival of the species (including procreation and raising children). It is also responsible for a range of automatic functions such as breathing, keeping our heart beating, regulation of the sleep cycle, the release of hormones and many other involuntary functions. All of these lobes work together. On a cellular level, neurons are found in all of the lobes of the brain. They work together to create our consciousness and enable the automatic functions of our body. Let's explore these neurons in more detail.

How Neurons Communicate

It is estimated that there are around a hundred billion neurons in a human brain. Give or take a few billion. No one has ever sat and counted every neuron. Not that we can blame anyone with the numbers involved. Just imagine being given that job! I wouldn't want to be *that* person.

Neurons communicate through electrical impulses and chemicals. Here is the process of neuron communication:

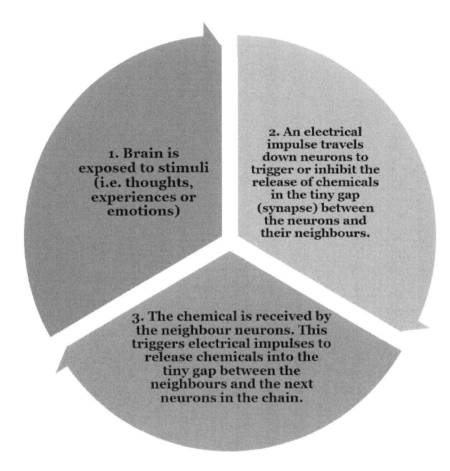

1. Brain is exposed to stimuli (i.e. thoughts, experiences or emotions).

2. An electrical impulse travels down neurons to trigger or inhibit the release of chemicals in the tiny gap (synapse) between the neurons and their neighbours.

3. The chemical is received by the neighbour neurons. This

triggers electrical impulses to release chemicals into the tiny gap between the neighbours and the next neurons in the chain.

Neurons communicate between each other super-fast. Each neuron is thought to fire chemicals or signals 5-50 times every second. That's a minimum of 18,000 signals every hour, per neuron (of which there are billions). That means at any one time there are zillions of signals being transmitted around your brain.

Understanding the chemicals transmitted between the neurons are essential to understanding the mechanics of the mind, along with how they influence mental health and mental illness. Let's look at the chemical players.

The Chemical Players

All of these chemicals are neurotransmitters, meaning that they transmit messages between the neurons as explained above. Here are our chemical players:

Serotonin - The happiness chemical. Makes you feel happy and content. It is made in the brain.

Dopamine - The motivation chemical. It not only motivates you, but makes you feel good. It is made in the brain.

Dopamine motivates you to seek out things you need for your individual and species survival. Such as food, water and sex. It does this by operating a reward pathway. When your brain gets whatever the dopamine has motivated you to seek out, it stimulates the release of more dopamine across the lobes of the brain. This dopamine makes you feel *really* good. This rewards the behaviour and makes you more likely to repeat it.

Never underestimate just *how good* dopamine can make you feel. Dopamine and its reward pathway are thought to be the physiological cause of addictions to substances, ultimately destructive behaviours (such as gambling or over eating) and even the high you get following a good session of exercise at the gym.

Noradrenaline - The alert for danger chemical. This chemical is made in the two adrenal glands, that are located at the top of each kidney. Along with Cortisol it gets your body ready to Fight, Flight or Freeze.

Cortisol - The stress hormone. This chemical is made in the two adrenal glands, that are located at the top of each kidney. Along with Noradrenaline it gets your body ready to Fight, Flight or Freeze.

The Fight, Flight or Freeze Response
The fight, flight or freeze response is your brain and body's reaction to a threat or perceived threat. Your body has a number of responses in the Fight, Flight or Freeze response mode:

- Pupils dilate to take in more visual information.
- The production of saliva stops.
- Makes the bronchi in the lungs bigger so that more oxygen can be inhaled.
- Makes the heart beat faster to get more oxygen to where it is needed quicker.
- Increases glucose levels in the blood so that cells have the extra energy required.
- Decreases activity in the stomach, pancreas, intestines and bladder by reducing blood flow to these organs, as

none of these organs or systems are required for the immediate in-the-moment survival.

The entire fight, flight or freeze response is about getting your body ready to fight the threat or perceived threat, run from the threat or perceived threat (flight) or freeze in indecision. The freeze response is like a rabbit freezing in the headlights of a car.

This response worked great when humans weren't the dominant form of life and when we had predators that wished to kill and eat us. However it isn't as useful today.

Today this response kicks in too often, in everyday events that aren't a threat to our survival. Some examples of modern-day events that our brain perceives as threats and activates our Fight, Flight or Freeze response include:

- Being under pressure by a tight deadline at work.
- Public speaking.
- Sitting in a traffic jam.
- Getting a car parking ticket.
- Financial difficulties or job insecurity.
- Our own critical inner voice criticising us (see Part 2 - Empathy Through Lived Experience section of this book, chapter Rumination & Critical Inner Voice for more information).
- Social conflict - including arguments and heated discussions.
- Sitting exams.
- Organising a big social occasion - such as a wedding.
- Job interviews.

- Unexpected knocks on a door, unexpected notifications or messages on our phones.
- The News.
- Horror and psychological thriller films.
- People's comments on social media posts.

The list could go on and on. What's interesting your brain only needs to perceive a threat for the fight, flight or freeze response to activate. Even you quickly realise that it isn't a threat and reassure your mind, it's too late. Your neurons have already activated the response.

Looking at the examples above trying to fight, running away from or freezing in these situations would be completely unhelpful at best and at worst illegal and morally wrong.

I'm thinking about you trying to fight people interviewing you. I would safely bet, that if you did this, you would not get the job. Unless you were applying to be a champion boxer, but even then, they probably wouldn't appreciate you assaulting them when they'd invited you in for a little chat.

Another interesting consideration is that your brain doesn't know if the threat is right in front of you or a thousand miles away.

Let's take the example of reading the news. If you read about a volcano erupting, killing people and severely burning others, it is likely that your fight, flight or freeze response will activate. Even though the volcano might be thousands of miles away, in a country that you have never been to, so is absolutely no threat to you, your brain still responds.

Merely thinking about something can active the response.

Your response might have been triggered just by reading the example above. Check in with how you feel physically, mentally and emotionally to see if this was the case.

Back to the last of our chemical players...

Oxytocin - The love and caring hormone. It makes you bond with partners, want to have sex with them, get attached to offspring and enables empathy. It is made in the brain.

Everything as Fact

Your brain is like a sponge, meaning that everything it sees, smells, touches, tastes and hears your brain accepts as fact. Even when you consciously know something is a lie, unconsciously your brain takes it as a fact. It is a survival mechanism, there are no lies in nature. Lies are a very human concept. That is why need supportive relationships.

Abuse in relationships whether that be physical, verbal or both can change the structures and functioning of your brain. Ever heard that saying - if you hear something enough, you'll start to believe it? It couldn't be truer.

The Brain in Anxiety

In someone with anxiety their brain will have low levels of serotonin, dopamine and oxytocin. They will have high levels of noradrenaline and cortisol. Knowing this helps the symptoms of anxiety make sense. Symptoms including:

- Being on edge.
- Feelings of fear and impending doom.
- Chest pain and heart palpitations.
- Sweating.
- Nausea (feeling sick).
- Over reacting to perceived threats.

- Panic attacks.

Anxiety often comes from indecision and is often irrational. Someone with anxiety will feel overwhelmed and often be in freeze response of the fight, flight or freeze responses. A good way to reduce anxiety is to make a decision. First identify triggers for your anxiety. Then decided how you will deal with these triggers.

For example, say you are anxious about losing your job and what that will mean for you and your family. The best way to deal with this is to accept that losing your job is a possibility. But recognise that there are things that you can do to make this less likely (such as meeting your targets at work, having good relationships with your work colleagues, etc.).

Some circumstances are beyond your control. Say your employer is making cut backs. You can't control whom the company decides to make redundant. You can still do all the things listed above, but this doesn't guarantee that it won't be you who is made redundant. When it comes down to it - you have to either accept that there is a possibility you could lose your job and chose to stay where you are; or accept that the job insecurity is too much for you to accept and chose to start looking for other employment opportunities.

The Brain in Depression
In someone with depression their brain will have low levels of serotonin, dopamine and oxytocin. They will have high levels of noradrenaline and cortisol. Knowing this helps the symptoms of depression make sense. Symptoms including:

- Tiredness and exhaustion.

- Difficulty in getting to sleep or staying asleep.
- Loss of pleasure in life and in doing activities previously enjoyed.
- Low motivation to do anything.
- Reduced appetite with or without weight loss.
- Weight gain caused by poor diet.
- Slowed thinking, speaking or difficulty in concentrating.
- Angry outbursts, feeling constantly frustrated or irritable.

Both anxiety and depression have the same effect on the brain. It isn't no wonder that people often have mixed episodes containing symptoms of both anxiety and depression together.

The Brain with Suicidal Thinking

It is estimated that around 1 in 5 people (20% of the population) will have suicidal thoughts at some point in their lives. But why do they get these thoughts? What's going on in the brain? Let me explain.

High levels of cortisol caused by chronic stress is extremely damaging to your brain. High levels of cortisol over a prolonged period can disrupt communication between neurons, kill neurons and even cause shrinking of the brain. The brain knows it must lower the levels of cortisol and suicidal thoughts aim to do just that.

When a person decides that they are going to commit suicide, their levels of cortisol instantly begin to drop. This is because they no longer need to worry or be stressed about the things that they are, as they won't be around to have to deal with any of their problems.

The brain knows that high levels of cortisol is damaging to it, so suicidal thoughts are about the brain encouraging a decision to be made that begins to lower cortisol levels.

Of course the brain doesn't *really* want the person to commit suicide, it's just about lowering cortisol levels. The brain has lots of strategies to prevent people acting on their suicidal ideation. You can read more about suicide in Part 2 - Empathy Through Lived Experience, The 'S' Word - Suicide chapter of this book.

A Quick Note on Thiamine
The human brain has a brain-to-body mass of just 2%, yet requires 20% of the total energy created from food to operate normally. Thiamine (Vitamin B1) is used to convert carbohydrates into glucose so it can be used by the neurons in the brain as energy. Thiamine is essential for normal brain functioning.

Foods that contain good amounts of Thiamine include: asparagus, brown rice, cereals, eggs, fish, green peas, lean pork chops, oranges, seaweed, spinach, sunflower seeds, tofu, and yeast to name a few.

Thiamine is poorly absorbed in the human digestive system and we can only store small amounts in the liver for a relatively short period of time. This means that we need to eat lots of Thiamine on a regular basis in order to maintain good brain functioning.

Survival, Reproduction & Evolution

Our brain and our body are fundamentally designed for survival and reproduction. Unfortunately being happy and mentally healthy are not essential to survival and reproduction.

There is no specific time frame that evolution takes to happen. However evolution can take thousands, if not, tens of thousands of years to occur. Now just think how much life has changed for humans in the last couple of hundred years.

Our brain hasn't had chance to change to better suit modern life. With the pressures of modern life, it's no wonder that many people suffer with mental illnesses.

The descriptions above have been simplified to make the Neuroscience more accessible. It is based on current knowledge and current theories. This means that in the future, as we develop our understanding of Neuroscience, some of the above might be proven incorrect or we may come to think of things differently than described as above. This is unavoidable and to be expected.

What causes Mental Illness?

There is a long-standing debate as to whether mental illness is as a result of nature (biology) or nurture (environment). There's lots of research to indicate that mental illness tends to run in families. This suggests that mental illness is a result of genes in our DNA.

However there's equal amounts of research suggesting that nurture plays a vital role in the *risk* of developing a mental illness. Nurture includes:

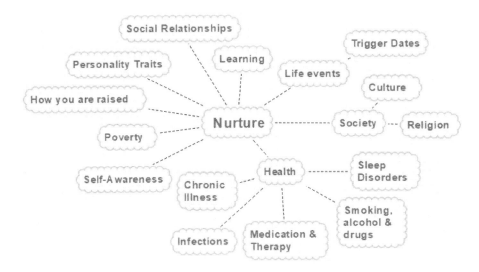

How you are raised is important because much of what we do is learned behaviour. What's important in how you are raised are the coping strategies you learn to deal with and overcome adversity.

Personality traits are important as these help to decide how you see and interact with the world. Some personality traits, like not wanting to ask for help can be unhelpful and potentially damaging to our mental health.

Social relationships can be positive or negative, but they are usually a mix of both. Being in codependent or abusive relationships can be extremely damaging to your mental health.

There's a wealth of evidences that demonstrates growing up or living in poverty has worse outcomes for both physical and mental health.

Self-awareness is vital to understanding our thoughts, feelings and behaviours. It is essential that we are aware of the state of our own mental health to prevent mental illness.

Our physical health is probably one of the most important things in our lives. People with chronic illnesses and sleep disorders have a much higher risk of developing mental illnesses. Infections can cause brain damage, which in turn can cause mental illness. Smoking, alcohol and drugs can all have a negative effect on our mental health. Medication and therapies can significantly improve our mental health.

Society, including culture and religion, have an influence in how we view mental health and illness and if we seek support or not.

Mental illness used to be a taboo topic in the UK. This caused people who were mentally ill to feel shame and guilt for being unwell. In the past some religions even viewed mental illness as a person being possessed by the devil or an evil spirit. These are two massive reasons why mental illness has traditionally had such a stigma attached to it. This has contributed to people feeling isolated, not being aware of support or accessing it and the high number of people committing suicide.

Learning is not about your level of academic achievement. It's about learning about mental health and illness and how to look after ourselves. We often learn this from our parents.

Unfortunately some of our parents might not be healthy role models. They will have learned off their parents and through life experience. It is likely that both your parents and grandparents grew up with mental health and mental illness as a taboo topics. So they are likely to just muddle through the best that they can, sometimes suffering with mental illnesses for years. This having a devastating impact on themselves and the people around them. Never accessing treatment that could transform them and their lives.

Traumatic life events can trigger mental illnesses. These life events could include: becoming homeless, abuse, violence, mental or emotional manipulation, bereavement of significant people in early life, divorce or relationship breakdown, financial difficulties, losing your job, neglect, loneliness and social isolation. The list could go on, but I'm sure that you get the idea.

Anniversaries of traumatic life events can also trigger mental illnesses or relapse - going from recovery back to having symptoms of mental illness again. To find out more about recovery, see the Treatments & Recovery chapter in this section of this book.

It is clear that mental illness is associated with a natural cause (genetics). But don't count your blessings if you haven't got anyone with mental illness in your family just yet. Nurture can increase the risk of developing mental illnesses in some cases and in other cases can trigger mental illnesses.

General Statistics for Mental Health in the UK

Here are some general statistics for mental health in the UK:

General Mental Health Statistics

1 in 4 will experience a mental health problem in any given year. (Time to Change, 2016)

Only one quarter of people with mental health problems seek treatment. (Mental Health Foundation, 2015)

The number of people seeking support around their mental health is increasing. (Mental Health Network NHS Confederation, 2016)

90% of people who are diagnosed with anxiety and depression are treated by their GP in primary care. (Mental Health Foundation, 2015)

Conditions in order of the number of people diagnosed: Mixed anxiety & depression, anxiety, self-harm, post traumatic stress disorder, depression, phobias, eating disorders, OCD and panic disorder. (Mind, 2016)

There were 121,499 admissions to mental health wards in the UK between 2013 and 2014. This reflected a 5.8% increase from the previous year. (Mental Health Foundation, 2015)

17 in every 100 people will have suicidal thoughts. (Mind, 2016)

There were 6,233 suicides in the UK in 2013. 78% were male. (Mental Health Foundation, 2015)

Statistics complied by Antony Simpson | www.antonysimpson.com

References

Time to Change (2016) *Myths/facts*, Last accessed: 4th December 2016.

Mental Health Foundation (2015) *Fundamental Facts About*

Mental Health 2015, Last accessed: 4th December 2016.

<u>Mind</u> (2016) *Mental health facts and statistics – Key facts and statistics on mental health problems and issues*, Last accessed: 4th December 2016.

<u>Mental Health Network NHS Confederation</u> (2016) *Factsheet March 2016 Key facts and trends in mental health 2016 update*, Last accessed: 4th December 2016.

A List of Famous People who have Experienced Mental Illness

Below is a list of famous people who have experienced mental health illnesses (in alphabetical order and by condition):

Anxiety and depression often coexist. Bipolar is characterised by episodes of mania which can include anxiety and episodes of depression. So although many of these people could fit under more than one mental illness, I have placed them in the condition that I feel bet fits.

Anxiety

- Charles Darwin, Naturalist & Geologist *[Deceased]*
- Heath Ledger, Actor *[Deceased]*
- Matt Haig, Author
- Vincent van Gogh, Painter *[Deceased]*

Bipolar

- Ben Stiller, Comedian & Actor
- Britney Spears, Singer
- Carrie Fisher, Advocate & Actress *[Deceased]*
- Catherine Zeta-Jones, Actress
- Isaac Newton, Mathematician & Physicist *[Deceased]*
- Russell Brand, Comedian

Depression

- Abraham Lincoln, Politician & Former President of the USA *[Deceased]*
- Alanis Morissette, Singer
- Anne Rice, Author

- Charles Dickens, Writer *[Deceased]*
- Denise Welch, Actress & Presenter
- Dolly Parton, Singer
- Drew Barrymore, Actress
- Emma Thompson, Writer & Actress
- George Michael, Singer *[Deceased]*
- Harrison Ford, Actor & Film Producer
- J.K Rowling, Author
- Jim Carrey, Comedian & Actor
- Kylie Minogue, Singer
- Diana Moutbatten-Windsor, Princess *[Deceased]*
- Robbie Williams, Singer
- Robin Williams, Comedian & Actor *[Deceased]*
- Ruby Wax, Comedian, Actress & Writer
- Stephen Fry, Presenter & Writer
- Stephen King, Author
- Trisha Goddard, Presenter
- Winston Churchill, Politician and Former Prime Minister of the UK *[Deceased]*

To anyone that is experiencing mental illness, you are among the great and the good.

Young People

A young person is any person aged between thirteen and twenty-one years old. They are in the adolescence stage of life:

Adolescence

The stage of adolescence or the teenage years starts around 12-13 years old and lasts until around 18-21 years old. The end of childhood and beginning of adolescence is marked by the start of puberty.

In adolescence the body and brain are going through massive changes. These changes mean that adolescents need more sleep and may well be found sleeping in till midday or later.

In the body, high levels of hormones rage creating physical changes, increasing emotional intensity and developing a fierce need for independence. The emotional intensity explains why adolescents are more likely to be rebellious in their thinking and actions.

Male physical changes in puberty include: growth of body hair (public, underarm, facial & legs), voice breaks – becoming deeper, Adam's apple becomes prominent, acne, penis growth, lowering of testis, growing taller and broader.

Female physical changes in puberty include: growth of breasts, menstrual cycle, growth of body hair (public, underarm & legs), acne, weight gain, change of body shape and growing taller.

In the brain, hormones make adolescents more likely to act on impulses and take risks. This explains why they are more likely to experiment with or use alcohol and/or drugs.

Both the body and brain make adolescents aware of those they feel sexually attracted to. They notice them. They want to get to know them. They ultimately want to have sex with them.

Adolescents may start to have sexual and/or romantic relationships.

An adolescent's thinking is egocentric – they are only or mostly concerned about themselves. This thinking explains a lot of adolescent behaviour including why they are so concerned about how they look.

Puberty takes around 4 years from the early signs to completion. As well as all the puberty changes, adolescents have the pressures of high school, including acceptance into peer groups and exams.

Why mention young people specifically?
These statistics explain why:

- *"20% of adolescents may experience a mental health problem in any given year.*
- *50% of mental health problems are established by age 14 and 75% by age 24.*
- *10% of children and young people (aged 5-16 years) have a clinically diagnosable mental problem, yet 70% of children and adolescents who experience mental health problems have not had appropriate interventions at a sufficiently early age."*

From: The Mental Health Foundation – Mental health statistics: children and young people, Last accessed: 06/10/18.

15 Lies That Depression Would Have You Believe

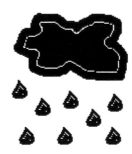

Here are 15 lies that depression would have you believe:

15. That it is bigger than you.

It's not. It just makes you think this so that it can keep in control of you.

14. That it would be better if you never left your bed/room/house again.

It wouldn't. You have so much to offer the world and you would miss out on so much if you never moved again. On days you feel like this practice self-compassion. Be kind but firm with yourself. Set yourself a small achievable goal. Force yourself into action to achieve this goal. Achieving a goal, no matter how small the goal is, will help you to feel better.

13. That you're a failure.

Firstly you're no failure. Failure comes by attempting to do or achieve things. Failure is no bad thing – you learn more through failure than you do success. Don't believe me? <u>watch this TED video where J.K. Rowling</u> talks about the benefits of her failures.

Depression likes to magnify experiences in your mind. It focuses on only the negative aspects of an experience. Most experiences are a mix of positives and negatives. Try to put experiences into perspective. Examine the positives. Try to practice balanced thinking and self-compassion.

12. That you'll never laugh again.

You will and often. People can and do recover from depression. Feeling okay doesn't mean that you're in recovery, starting to feel good again does. If you're just feeling okay, go and see your GP.

In recovery you will start to experience a number of long-lost emotions such as happiness, joy and elation. When you do, greet them as old friends and experience them fully.

11. That being physically, mentally and emotionally exhausted is a normal state of being.

It isn't. You might be sleeping for 18 hours and wake up still exhausted or you might be suffering with insomnia. But people usually have a stable amount of energy throughout the day and should sleep for a recommended 8 hours.

Depression is physically, mentally and emotionally exhausting, but if you go to your GP and get the right treatment things will improve.

10. That you're pathetic. That you have no right to feel the way you do. That you are a disappointment to all that know you.

Shame and guilt are two emotions that depression uses to try and control you. Let go of any shame and guilt you feel. Accept how you feel now and know that it is temporary, almost fleeting compared with your life. Be confident knowing that how you feel now will change with the passage of time.

9. That the physical, mental and emotional pain you feel is all that there is.

There's more to life pain. There's care, love, happiness, joy and so much more. Just hold on. You have experienced the more-than-pain emotions before and you will again.

8. That you can't do anything right or well enough.

My mum has lots of wisdom. She once said that all anyone can ask of you is that you try your best. Remember these words.

Put things into perspective. Ask yourself: What where your intentions? Did you kill anybody? No? Well then, it's not the end of the world.

7. That you are worthless.

You are unique. There has never been anyone exactly the same as you and there never will be. You are priceless and beyond value measures. Don't listen to this lie, instead remind yourself that you are special and remind yourself what makes you, you.

6. That you're going mad, mental or losing your mind.

No you're not. Your brain is just overwhelmed with cortisol – the stress hormone at the moment. Take a break and stop doing anything that you don't need to do. Practice relaxation techniques and be kind to yourself.

Remember that among the great and the good are people

who've experienced depression. Even at the height of their success.

5. That everything is too much effort. That just getting up and out of bed is too exhausting.

Set yourself a small goal each day and try your best to achieve it. The goal might be as tiny as having a bath, calling someone for a quick chat, changing your bedding or going for a short walk.

4. That your soul or higher self is being destroyed.

Your soul or higher self has survived several lifetimes and the accompanying reincarnation processes. It can and **will** survive depression. Depression is insignificant in comparison to the challenges your soul or higher self has already experienced.

3. That everything is hopeless.

You may feel this way, but it is not and will never be hopeless. According to The Royal College of Psychiatrists people can and do fully recover from depression.

2. That life isn't worth living.

Here's a plea from the heart: darling you might feel this way now, but how you feel will change. *If you are feeling suicidal please visit your nearest A&E Department for crisis support immediately.*

1. That you'll never be happy again.

You will. It will just take the right treatment and recovery time.

Assessment & Diagnosis

Assessment for mental illness depends on who is doing the assessment.

General Practitioners (GPs) will use the Generalised Anxiety Disorder (GAD-7) assessment to assess for anxiety and the Patient Health Questionnaire (PHQ-9) to assess for depression. They may also undertake a physical examination, bloods and other investigations to rule out any underlying physical causes of symptoms.

The Crisis Team assess people who are having a mental illness crisis usually in Accident & Emergency Departments. A crisis might involve suicidal thoughts, self-harm, overdoses, hallucinations or someone having lost touch with reality.

Assessment is usually undertaken by a Community Psychiatric Nurse (CPN). The assessment is usually about dealing with the immediate crisis, assessing risk of harm to self and others and coming up with a care plan. Long-term diagnosis is not made during a crisis.

Inpatients admitted on a mental health ward are under the care of a named Consultant Psychiatrist. There is usually a period of patient observation before any diagnosis is made or treatments are given. It can be a scary experience being admitted to a mental health ward. But sometimes it is the key to getting the right diagnosis and treatment.

The Community Mental Health Team have a comprehensive assessment. The assessment includes:

- Family history of mental illness.

- Details of symptoms (duration, frequency, impact on activities of daily living).
- Mental illness history, including details of past crisis'.
- How the patient presents and communicates.
- Details of previous treatments tried (medications and talking therapies).
- Personal history: occupation.
- Caring responsibilities and support networks.
- Physical illnesses or health problems.
- Treatment compliance for both physical and mental illnesses.
- Smoking status, alcohol use and drug use.
- Sexual health.
- Any legal issues.
- Identification of any Safeguarding issues.
- Any other professional involvements and reason for these involvements.
- A risk assessment.

The assessment usually takes more than 45 minutes. From this assessment, a care plan is developed. This care plan may include regular reviews with a Consultant Psychiatrist and regular sessions with a Psychologist and/or CPN.

Psychiatrists may use the Diagnostic and Statistical Manual of Mental Disorders (DSM-5) to help them make their diagnosis. A diagnosis may take years to make and there is always the chance of a misdiagnosis.

Treatments for the symptoms of mental illness are much quicker than the diagnosis process. You can read more about available treatments in the Treatments & Recovery chapter of this book.

A List of Common Conditions

Here is a list of some common mental health conditions in alphabetical order:

Addictions – Alcohol, Drugs, Sex, Gambling, etc.

Addictions are compulsive habits or behaviours that are usually damaging to the individual and their families. They maybe physical and/or psychological in nature.

If the addictions are physical in nature - such as alcohol and heroin, users get to the point where they use the drug to feel normal, rather than to get high. Stopping these drugs suddenly and without professional help can result in the user becoming physically and mentally unwell and can be life threatening. For example, suddenly stopping alcohol, if you are physically dependent, carries the risks of seizures and possibly death.

The harms caused by addictions include: damage to physical, mental and emotional health; finding it difficult to do activities of daily living - such as eating, bathing and sleeping; breakdown in relationships; loss of contact with children; lying; loosing or being unable to maintain a job; turning to crime to fund the addictions; problems created by things said and done when intoxicated; the risk of overdosing with the potential for death.

According to NHS Choices certain people are more at risk of developing an addiction:

"You're more at risk of developing an addiction if:
– other members of your family have addiction problems
– you experienced stress or abuse while growing up
– you have mental health problems"

(From: <u>NHS Choices</u>, Last Accessed on 28th December 2014)

People can and do overcome addictions. In order to do so, they must want to. Then they must address the root causes of their addictions. After that, they need to find different strategies to manage their thoughts, emotions and behaviours and put these into place.

The right support is essential. In the UK, every geographical area has community alcohol and drug treatment service. People are usually referred to these services by their GP. Many people also find mutual aid groups, such as Alcoholics Anonymous (AA) or Narcotics Anonymous (NA) useful.

For more information visit: Talk to Frank, DrugScope, Drink Aware & Gamblers Anonymous.

Anxiety
"Anxiety is a feeling of unease, such as worry or fear, that can be mild or severe.

Everyone has feelings of anxiety at some point in their life. For example, you may feel worried and anxious about sitting an exam or having a medical test or job interview. During times like these, feeling anxious can be perfectly normal.

However, some people find it hard to control their worries. Their feelings of anxiety are more constant and can often affect their daily life.

Anxiety is the main symptom of several conditions, including panic disorder, phobias, post-traumatic stress disorder and social anxiety disorder (social phobia)."

(From: NHS Choices, Last Accessed on 28th December 2014)

A friend of mine appeared to be one of the most laid-back people that I knew. Once he was away on holiday with his wife and two children. A place with sun, sea and sand, that they are familiar with as they holiday there a couple of times a year.

He was relaxing by the pool, topping up his tan, when he suddenly got a sharp stabbing pain in his chest. He felt like he couldn't breath and everything around him started to spin. In absolute terror, he thought that he was having a heart attack and was going to die. He called out to his wife who called an ambulance.

He was swiftly taken to hospital. At the hospital, after doing a range of tests and investigations, they gave him his diagnosis: he'd had a panic attack.

Panic attacks often come out of the blue. The good news is that although panic attacks are frightening, they usually only last a maximum of 20 minutes. A helpful tip for a person experiencing a panic attack is to focus on their breathing or something else - like focusing on the feel of the floor under their feet, until the panic subsides.

My friend is now more open and honest with everyone about the things he is worried about.

Some people may have one panic attack and never have another. Some many get intermittent panic attacks, others get regular panic attacks. For those who get regular panic attacks they are able to identify triggers and manage or avoid these triggers.

For more information visit: Anxiety UK & No Panic.

Bipolar

Bipolar used to be called manic depression. Bipolar is associated mood swings, including highs (manic episodes), lows (depressive episodes) and mixed mood states (where both high and low symptoms are present at the same time).

The exact frequency and severity of mood swings varies massively depending upon the individual and environmental factors.

"If you have bipolar disorder, you will have periods or episodes of:
– depression – where you feel very low and lethargic
– mania – where you feel very high and overactive (less severe mania is known as hypomania)

Symptoms of bipolar disorder depend on which mood you are experiencing. Unlike simple mood swings, each extreme episode of bipolar disorder can last for several weeks (or even longer), and some people may not experience a 'normal' mood very often."

(From: NHS Choices, Last Accessed on 28th December 2014)

There are different types of Bipolar including:

- Bipolar 1 - To be diagnosed with this type, you must have had a manic episode that resulted you being hospitalised. If untreated manic episodes last around 3-6 months and depressive episodes last around 6-12 months.
- Bipolar 2 - There's a more prevalence of depressive episodes in Bipolar type 2. They have hypomanic episodes, but not severe manic episodes.
- Cyclothymia - This is a form of Bipolar where symptoms are said to be less severe. Manic, depressive and mixed

episodes can all happen. Some people call this *a mild form of bipolar.* But for those with this diagnosis, it is anything *but* mild. 50% of people diagnosed with this form of Bipolar go on to be re-diagnosed later with either Bipolar 1 or Bipolar 2.

In an episode of mania or depression it can lead to psychosis. Psychosis is losing touch with reality, having hallucinations or delusions.

It is estimated that 1 million people in the UK are diagnosed with Bipolar. What is clear is that the mood swings in Bipolar have a devastating impact the individual, their functioning and on those around them.

Treatment usually involves an anti-psychotic mood stabiliser (to balance out the highs and lows), sometimes an anti-depressant (to relieve symptoms of depressive episodes) and talking therapies. Treatments and Recovery are discussed in further detail the next chapter of this book.

For more information visit: Bipolar UK.

Bereavement
Bereavement is a normal reaction to the death of a loved one.

"After a death you may initially feel shocked, numb, guilty, angry, afraid and full of pain. These feelings may change to feelings of longing, sadness, loneliness – even hopelessness and fear about the future."

(From: Cruse Bereavement Care – Has someone died? Restoring Hope, Last Accessed on 28th December 2014)

The Grief Cycle developed by Kubler-Ross, explains the emotions people go through during a bereavement.

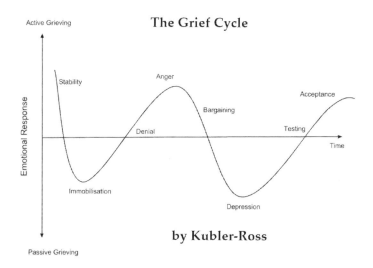

1. Stability - This is the first stage of the cycle before the death takes place.

2. Immobilisation - Can also be called shock. This is more commonly experienced in unexpected deaths.

3. Denial - This is about trying to emotionally avoid the fact of the death and about how it will change your life.

4. Anger -This is often experienced in unexpected deaths, such as accidents or sudden undiagnosed medical conditions that lead to death. There is a feeling of unfairness and *why did they have to die?*

5. Bargaining - This is the start of coming to terms with the loss.

6. Depression - This is being low in mood specifically triggered

by the death of someone.

7. Testing - This is about thinking about how to adapt to the loss of someone. Perhaps trying to get back to some sense of a normality.

8. Acceptance - This is accepting that the death has happened and that life has changed. It is about realising that life goes on. Understanding that your love for deceased will stay in your heart and finding a way to continue with your life.

People can go forwards and backwards on The Grief Cycle, as well as getting stuck at particular stages.

Everyone's journey through grief is unique. They might not experience all of the emotions above. Equally, when they grief for the next person, their experience will be different.

People may go through the cycle above quite quickly or quite slowly. There is no time limit on grief.

For more information visit: NHS Choices – Bereavement & Cruse Bereavement Care.

Depression
"Depression is a real illness with real symptoms, and it's not a sign of weakness or something you can 'snap out of' by 'pulling yourself together'...

Depression affects people in different ways and can cause a wide variety of symptoms.

They range from lasting feelings of sadness and hopelessness, to losing interest in the things you used to enjoy and feeling very tearful. Many people with depression also have symptoms of anxiety.

There can be physical symptoms too, such as feeling constantly tired, sleeping badly, having no appetite or sex drive, and complaining of various aches and pains.

The severity of the symptoms can vary. At its mildest, you may simply feel persistently low in spirit, while at its most severe depression can make you feel suicidal and that life is no longer worth living."

(From: NHS Choices, Last Accessed on 28th December 2014)

For more information visit: Depression Alliance.

Eating Disorders

People with eating disorders have an unhealthy relationship with food. This unhealthy relationship leads to dramatically eating less or more, or vomiting food recently eaten in a process known as purging.

People with eating disorders have body dysmorphic disorder. The disorder is characterised by people having an obsession on how their body looks and a view that it is deeply flawed or disgusting. These thoughts and associated emotions are so constant and overpowering that they find it difficult to think about anything else.

Common symptoms include: rapid weight loss or gain, a sudden obsession with calories, excessive exercising, an aversion to eating with others, an aversion to mirrors and possible frequent visits to the toilet during or just after a meal.

"Types of eating disorders
"Eating disorders include a range of conditions that can affect someone physically, psychologically and socially. The most common eating disorders are:

– anorexia nervosa – when someone tries to keep their weight as low as possible, for example by starving themselves or exercising excessively
– bulimia – when someone tries to control their weight by binge eating and then deliberately being sick or using laxatives (medication to help empty their bowels)
– binge eating – when someone feels compelled to overeat

Some people, particularly young people, may be diagnosed with an eating disorder not otherwise specified (EDNOS). This is means you have some, but not all, of the typical signs of eating disorders such as anorexia or bulimia."

(From: NHS Choices, Last Accessed on 28th December 2014)

For more information visit: beat.

Obsessive Compulsive Disorder (OCD)
OCD is a condition were people's mind are obsessed with completing repeated behaviours or have repetitive and intrusive thoughts.

OCD symptoms are on a spectrum from mild to very severe. Many people joke about being OCD or on the spectrum. This only minimises the recognition of the symptoms of severe end of the spectrum.

The thoughts and behaviours on the severe end of the spectrum can be debilitating and take over people's life.

"Some people with OCD may spend an hour or so a day engaged in obsessive-compulsive thinking and behaviour, but for others the condition can completely take over their life."

(From: NHS Choices, Last Accessed on 28th December 2014)

For more information visit: <u>OCD Action</u> & <u>Mind – Obsessive Compulsive Disorder (OCD)</u>.

Schizophrenia

"Schizophrenia is a long-term mental health condition that causes a range of different psychological symptoms, including:
– hallucinations – hearing or seeing things that do not exist
– delusions – unusual beliefs not based on reality which often contradict the evidence
– muddled thoughts based on the hallucinations or delusions
– changes in behaviour

Doctors often describe schizophrenia as a psychotic illness. This means sometimes a person may not be able to distinguish their own thoughts and ideas from reality."

(From: <u>NHS Choices</u>, Last Accessed on 28th December 2014)

For more information visit: <u>Rethink: Schizophrenia</u>.

Seasonal Affective Disorder (SAD)

SAD is a type of depression that occurs during the winter months when there is less sun light. Sun light provides Vitamin D, which improves mood.

Signs and symptoms of SAD include:

- Low mood - feeling that everything is pointless and loss of pleasure in what should be pleasurable activities.
- Lack of energy that maybe accompanied by sleeping more or less or insomnia.
- Irritability.
- Feelings of guilt and shame.
- An increase in the frequency and volume of the critical inner voice.

- Weight gain or loss. Changes to appetite.

Stress

Stress is when we feel under too much mental or emotional pressure. There are two forms of stress, acute stress and chronic stress. Acute stress is stress on a short-term basis. Chronic stress is stress on a long-term basis.

Stress can be caused by a range of experiences in life including: doing too much or having too much work to do at work, difficult relationships - with family, friends or partners, money problems, health problems, difficult emotions and recurrent worrying.

Signs and symptoms of stress include:

- Irritability or being overly defensive.
- Difficulties with memory or concentration.
- Muscle tension (particularly in the upper back and shoulders).
- Headaches.
- Anxiety or worrying about how much you have to do and what you didn't get done that day.
- Being upset, tearful or feeling downtrodden.
- Interrupted sleep.
- A sense of dread.
- Feeling neglected, isolated or lonely.
- Changes to eating patterns and amounts.
- High blood pressure.

"Once the pressure or threat has passed, your stress hormone levels will usually return to normal. However, if you're constantly under stress, these hormones will remain in your

body, leading to the symptoms of stress."

(From: <u>NHS Choices</u>, Last Accessed on 28th December 2014).

The best way to deal with stress is to have good coping strategies and fill up your Well of Resilience (see Part 3 - Life Hacks, The Well of Resilience chapter).

Chronic stress can lead to depression and anxiety. So it's good to identify the causes of stress and deal with them early on.

For more information visit: <u>Mind – How to manage stress</u> & <u>Mental Health Foundation – Stress</u>.

Post-Traumatic Stress Disorder (PTSD)
PTSD is a type of anxiety and stress disorder caused by witnessing or being involved in emotionally traumatic events.

PTSD is common in those who have experienced childhood abuse (including physical, emotional, neglect and sexual abuse), domestic violence, rape, severe accidents, natural disasters, terrorist attacks or are military veterans (around 6% of UK army personal are diagnosed with PTSD).

Someone with PTSD may have flashbacks or nightmares of the event(s) that caused their PTSD. They may feel extremely anxious. They may try to forget the events and associated feelings through self-medication. Self-medication could include the use of alcohol, drugs or prescription painkillers.

Treatments & Recovery

I want to write about treatment options and discuss recovery.

Treatment Options

Treatment options vary depending on the individual, but may include:

- Medications – such as antidepressants, anti-anxiety, mood stabilisers, anti-psychotics or other medications to manage symptoms (such as sedatives in the short-term to help a person sleep if they have been suffering with insomnia). People may be given one medication or a combination of different medications to take.
- Talking Therapies – such as Counselling, Cognitive Behavioural Therapy (CBT) and MCBT (Mindfulness-based Cognitive Behaviour Therapy).
- A combination of medication(s) and talking therapies.
- Meditation or mindfulness.

Treatments maybe prescribed by a GP or by the GP making a referral on to other services. For example, the GP may refer onto services that provide Talking Therapies or to the Community Mental Health Team. For the majority of people, they will be treated in their community.

Only people with severely poor mental health, usually where they are deemed a risk to themselves or others, will be treated as an inpatient on a hospital ward. This hospital admission might be on a voluntary basis or by sectioning someone under the Mental Health Act (1983).

Medication

People with mental illnesses have mixed views about medications. Some people seem to be against the use of medications for managing symptoms.

Often they will boast about changes to their diet, taking food supplements and changes to lifestyle (such as going to the gym regularly) to manage their symptoms of their mental illness. They seem completely against the use of medications, but it is difficult to establish why they feel this way.

It is likely that their views are due to the stigma associated with mental illness, fear of side effects from medication(s), or mythical tales of people who have had severe side effects on medications.

I say mythical tales as people often don't know the person the tales are about. The tales are usually told to them by family or friends.

Medications can have side effects. These side effects range from very mild to severe.

The best way to view the use of medications is this: Your brain is an organ in your body. Like any other organ it can get sick. Medications help manage the symptoms and help in the recovery process.

If someone had a bacterial chest infection, they wouldn't debate taking antibiotics to treat it. No one would advise them not to take the antibiotics prescribed by their GP. They would take the medication to help manage the symptoms and to help in the recovery process. The same way of thinking should be applied to medicines for mental illnesses.

Talking Therapies

General Counselling, Cognitive Behaviour Therapy (CBT) and MCBT (Mindfulness-based Cognitive Behaviour Therapy) are the three most common forms of Talking Therapies.

General counselling aims to support people to explore their own emotions, problems and come up with their own solutions to their problems. A Counsellor may work with someone on a one-to-one basis or in a small group.

Counselling can be delivered in person, on the telephone or online. The number of counselling sessions should be based on the needs of the individual.

Counselling sessions on the National Health Service (NHS) are often limited by time per session and number of sessions.

CBT & MCBT is more structured than general counselling. CBT/MCBT examines thoughts, emotions, physical sensations and actions.

In CBT the theory is that our thoughts influence our emotions, physical sensations and actions. By changing what we think and the way in which we think, we change our emotions, physical sensations and actions. This is what the therapy focuses on. It also involves challenging any negative beliefs someone has about themselves or others.

MCBT adds mindfulness to CBT. Mindfulness is the practice of being fully present in the here and now. Noticing the details with your five senses:

- What do you see?
- What do you hear?

- What can you smell?
- What can you feel (this could be the clothes on your skin or what you can touch with your hands)?
- And if applicable, what can you taste?

Whenever your mind drifts away from the five senses, you gently bring it back to focus on the senses. The idea is to practice mindfulness until it becomes habit. Once it starts to become habit, mindfulness stops wondering thoughts, makes people more present in the here and now, and increases awareness of self and others. Mindfulness increases people's ability to accept things as they are with the minimum amount of intruding thoughts or feelings.

One of the key differences between general counselling and CBT/MCBT is that in counselling sessions someone may discuss their past. Whereas CBT/MCBT focus on the now.

There are other talking therapies, including: motivational interviewing, solution focused therapy and goal setting.

With motivational interviewing the Counsellor aims to motivation a person to make changes in their lives.

Solution focused therapy is solution-focused. Once the problem is identified, it isn't given any more time or energy. Instead the time and energy goes into trying to find solutions. A key belief using this type of talking therapy is that the person with the problem also has the solution inside them. It's the Counsellor's job to help the person find their own solutions from within.

Goal setting is about setting realistic and achievable goals. It involves breaking goals down into a series of small tasks for the person to complete in order for them to achieve their goals.

The Most Effective Treatment

Research suggests that the best and most effective treatment are a combination of the right medications and talking therapies.

Meditation or Mindfulness

Meditation or mindfulness should be used in combination with medication(s) and/or talking therapies. Both mediation and mindfulness are skills. To get good at any skill you must practice them often. The basics of mindfulness have been discussed above.

The aims of meditation are to give clarity and a state of calmness. There's no right or wrong way to meditate. The focuses of mediation sessions can include:

- Clearing you mind of all thoughts and emotions, so that your mind is essentially a black empty space.
- Focusing on a single thought, feeling, event or challenge. This is usually to learn, increase your self-awareness, to check in with yourself and open your mind up to possible solutions to any problems you might be having.
- Focusing on a visualisation. Your brain can't tell the difference between a visualisation and reality. So if you visualise yourself on a beach with the tide coming slowly in and out, the heat of the sun penetrating your muscles and easing the tension, you will to start to physically and mentally relax. The key to visualisations is that you must imagine what you would see, hear, smell, touch and taste.

When someone first starts meditation or mindfulness their mind will wonder. The person just needs to gently, without any internal judgement or criticism, bring their mind back to the exercise. It is recommended that someone starts with 5 minute sessions, setting an alarm so that they know when the session is over. From there slowly building up the length and frequency of the sessions.

Recovery

This is what the Mental Health Foundation writes about recovery:

"In mental health, recovery does not always refer to the process of complete recovery from a mental health problem in the way that we may recover from a physical health problem.

What is recovery?
For many people, the concept of recovery is about staying in control of their life despite experiencing a mental health problem. Professionals in the mental health sector often refer to the 'recovery model' to describe this way of thinking.

Putting recovery into action means focusing care on supporting recovery and building the resilience of people with mental health problems, not just on treating or managing their symptoms.

There is no single definition of the concept of recovery for people with mental health problems, but the guiding principle is hope – the belief that it is possible for someone to regain a meaningful life, despite serious mental illness.

Recovery is often referred to as a process, outlook, vision, conceptual framework or guiding principle."

(From: Mental Health Foundation, Last Accessed: 31st December 2014.)

I have recovered from past episodes of mental illness, as have other people that I know. Although I have recovered from these episodes, I know that I need to keep a close eye on my mental health.

Some people have more difficulty with recovery than others. My hope is that as medical research improves our understanding of how the brain functions and that this will improve treatments of mental health conditions. This would mean people with mental illnesses would suffer less, that it will be easier for them to recover and that they will spend more of their lives in recovery.

Everyone's idea of recovery is different. But it is a journey. You are *not* going to wake up one day recovered. Anyone who tells you otherwise is either totally unaware of what recovery is or is lying. Being in recovery may include:

- Feeling happy again.
- Being able to do activities of daily living again.
- Returning to work or employment.
- Being educated about your mental illness and how to stay well.
- Being active in the community.
- Supporting and helping others.
- Finding your life purpose.
- Reconnecting with your family and friends.
- Living life according to your values.

- Effectively managing your triggers.
- Feeling fully present in the moment.
- Working towards/achieving your goals.
- Being self-aware so that you spot any deterioration in your mental health.
- Building self-care into your life.
- Feeling passionate, purposeful and learning something new.

The Drama Triangle

The Drama Triangle is a psychological and behavioural theory developed in the late 60s by Stephen Karpman. Although a theory, many people find they relevant to situations and relationships that they experience everyday.

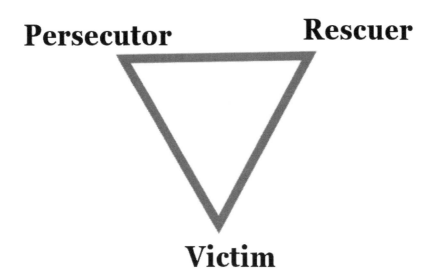

The Drama Triangle

Persecutor   **Rescuer**

Victim

by Stephen Karpman

The theory has three roles: victim, persecutor and rescuer.

The victim is powerless. No matter the situation. They

perceive they have no choices and that the odds are stacked against them. They like to complain to anyone that will listen. They generally like their role. They will be obstructive and defensive to people offering advice around changes they can make to improve their lives. There will always be an excuse as to why they can't make changes to their lives.

Victims take no responsibility for their actions or choices or the consequences of their actions or choices. Victims need a persecutor and usually a rescuer, so they will often draw people into situations to play these roles.

Persecutors can be another individual (such as the victim's boss at work), a group of individuals or organisations (such as Police or Government).

Genuine persecutors like to blame the victim, make victim's feel bad and are inflexible when dealing with the victim. Persecutors usualy treat the victim differently than they do others.

However not all people that are labelled as persecutors actually are. Just because the victim's perception is that they are a persecutor doesn't make it true.

Rescuers are generally kind people who try to help the victim out.

Rescuers have many motivations behind their actions. Motivations include: feeling that it is their role (as a parent/grandparent/carer), a craving for others to like and accept them, empathising with the victim, having been in the same situation as the victim in the past, having low self-esteem that is boosted by doing something good and feelings of guilt or shame that they know they'll experience if they don't help.

The victims, persecutors and rescuers are all acting on emotions. The drama triangle is usually played out on a unconscious level, with those playing the different roles completely unaware that they are doing so. The best way to know if you're in a drama triangle or are being drawn into one is to be self-aware.

There are two key concepts to get your head around with The Drama Triangle:

1. Victims will always try to bring you into a situation to play a role. Be wary of anyone that wants you to play a specific role or respond in a specific way rather than being yourself.
2. It doesn't have to be this way. If all involved start thinking with logic, rather than relying on emotions, and took personal responsibility for their actions this triangle would breakdown and dissolve away. Unfortunately victims find this incredibly difficult to do.

The Cycle of Life

Life is a cycle. It has stages or distinct periods, associated with age and these ages are also associated with key events. Understanding the cycle of life and where you are can help to explain your thoughts, feelings and behaviours. Everyone who lives a full life cycle will goes through each of these stages. They are:

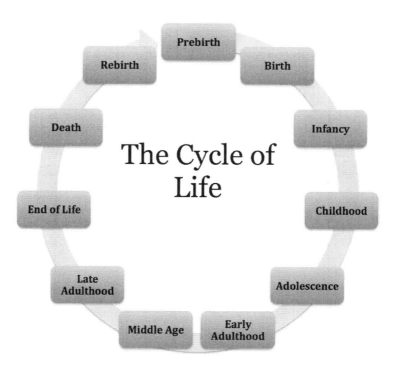

Image from: www.antonysimpson.com | Copyright © Antony Simpson, 2018.

Prebirth

There is some debate between Scientists, Doctors, Religious Leaders and Philosophers about when human life actually begins. Some say it begins at conception or fertilisation (generally most Religious Leaders), whereas Scientists and Doctors in the UK state that human life begins once a fertilised egg has implanted its self into the uterus wall, based on medical research and legal judgements.

Whichever you believe to be correct, this stage of life goes from 0-40 weeks. In this time you grow from a single cell into an embryo (from day four of fertilisation to week eight of pregnancy) and then into a foetus (from week eight of pregnancy until birth). Your mother will go through the three trimesters of pregnancy. You will be called a baby from birth.

Birth

You come into this world as a baby that is fully dependent on your mother, father and/or other carers to meet your needs for: milk, hygiene, warmth, sleep, safety, stimulation and love (emotional attachment and bonding). This is a period of rapid physical growth.

By 3-6 months old you will need to be weaned on to solid foods to satisfy your hunger and to give you enough nutrients to continue this rapid period of physical growth. Between 6-9 months old you will begin exploring your physical environment by crawling.

By 1 year old you begin to walk and enter into the infancy stage of your life cycle.

Infancy

In this stage you learn through exploration and play. This stage is usually between the ages of 1 to 5 years. You develop in all sorts of ways including:

- Physically – you continue to grow, develop gross and fine motor skills.

- Cognitively – you develop your ability to solve basic problems and begin to develop your imagination.
- Language – You learn to communicate verbally through speech. You will go from knowing a handful of words to hundreds.
- Socially – You learn to parallel play, to share and social rules.
- Emotionally – You learn to identify what you feel and eventually to emotionally regulate yourself.
- Moral – You begin to notice what is perceived as right and wrong.
- In infancy, a significant phase for most parents or carers is the terrible twos. To call it the *terrible twos* is a bit deceptive though, as it starts from around 18 months and can carry on until the infant is 3 and a half years old.

You say 'No' often and temper tantrum if you don't get your way. In the *terrible twos* you are learning what the boundaries are, what you can get away with and how to regulate your feelings of frustration and anger when you don't get what you want.

Childhood

Personality begins to develop in childhood, including likes and dislikes. Childhood starts at around 5 years old and ends around 12 years old (its ending being marked by the beginning of puberty).

As well as your personality developing, you become much less dependent on your parents or carers for your basic needs. You start structured learning at school, which leads to a more structured way of thinking. But conversely you are able to think abstractly.

You increase the number social relationships you have by making friends. You continue to grow – both physically and intellectually and continue to develop new skills. You may master some of these new skills. You have things that make you curious about the world and things that don't. You have passions and interests.

Adolescence

See previous chapter on Young People.

Early Adulthood

18-40 years old is the Early Adulthood stage of the cycle of life. Adults are physically fully grown and must use the life skills that they acquired in earlier stages to fend for themselves. In these few short years a lot happens in life.

You may move out of home; you may go to college and/or university; you may learn to drive a car; you go out into the world of work and start your career; you may make a commitment to a partner through marriage; you may end a relationship through divorce; you may buy your own home; you may have children of your own; you may travel; you may become more involved in community activities.

You feel enthusiastic about making your mark on the world. You continue to develop your passions and interests. Days, months and years pass quickly by at this stage of your life. You have little time to contemplate your life and the past choices you have made.

Middle Age

Contemplation is the keyword in middle age, which starts around 45 years old until around 65 years old. Physical signs of ageing are present and women will have started the menopause. People talk about having a midlife crisis in this stage.

You think about your life and if you are happy with it or not. You may feel that your life is stale and stagnant. This contemplation can cause you to make major changes in your life. However you may be perfectly content with your life and choose to continue on without making any major changes.

In this stage of your life you may need to care for your now elderly parents. You will have attended christenings, birthdays, weddings and funerals. You will have met and know people at all stages of the cycle of life.

Late Adulthood

Retirement from work will have occurred by the time a person reaches late adulthood. Late adulthood is a stage for people aged 65-75 years old. By this point people should have gained a wealth of wisdom as a result of life experiences.

You physically and mentally begin to slow down. You may regularly replay memories from your past.

End of Life

At the end of life the reflection continues. Most people will be 76+ years old. If people are happy with their life, they will feel satisfaction. However some people will have regrets.

People regret things like: not spending enough time with family and friends, not being the best parent/grandparent that they could have been, not having taken enough risks and playing it safe.

Death

According to The Office of National Statistics, the average life expectancy for a man is 79 years old and for a woman 83 years old, so for most death comes between 79-83 years old.

Your family and friends will grief for the loss of you in their lives. Hopefully they will celebrate your life as well.

Rebirth

Rebirth hasn't been scientifically proven at this point. But several religions and spiritual paths believe in reincarnation or rebirth. This is where you would be reborn either as another human or as an animal after death.

Even more fascinating is that some religions and spiritual paths believe that it is your *choice* to be reincarnated or remain on an astral/energy-based plane of existence.

The Future

A healthier lifestyle including: a good diet, regular exercise, not smoking, not drinking alcohol, not misusing substances, working/living in better environments with conditions that promote good health; along with ever-improving healthcare and technology will extend the life cycles of current and future people.

This extended life cycle may mean that in the future some of the ages people enter the stages stated above will change.

The Secrets to Self-Awareness

The Secrets to:

Self-Awareness

Self-awareness is about understanding more about you. It's about being aware of your thoughts, feelings, ego, knowledge, skills, experiences, relationships, communication, strengths & weaknesses, drives, values and behaviours in a situation. Self-awareness isn't something you do just once or occasionally. It should be an on-going day by day, hour by hour, moment by moment task.

There are numerous benefits to being more self-aware. A good example is that you can use self-awareness to change how you respond to different discussions and events to get better outcomes. It is just about you being aware of yourself and how you influence others. Nobody can be self-aware at all times, but you can make yourself more self-aware.

How do you become more self-aware? Here's my suggestions, based on research online and my own experiences:

1. Observation
Observe everything going on around you. Including yourself and how you interact with others.

2. Reflection
Reflect on just about everything. It could be a past experience, or reflecting on something you've learned or

read. Consider:

- Who? What? Why? How? When?
- What were your thought?
- What were your feelings?
- What were your behaviours?
- How did others behave?
- What do you think others wanted to gain?
- What outcome did you want? Did you get it? If not, what could you do differently?
- What did you learn? How can you use this learning in the future?

People have lots of different ways of reflecting. Some good ideas include: meditation, keeping a daily journal and counselling sessions (using the counsellor as a sounding board).

Two important things about reflection:
1. You've got to practice reflection to get good at it.
2. It has to become a regular behavioural habit.

3. Balanced Thinking
When observing or reflecting ensure that your thinking is balanced. When it comes to ourselves, we are often too critical and only see the negatives. Be fair and kind to yourself. Recognise both the positives and negatives.

4. Develop Your Emotional Intelligence
Emotional intelligence is about being able to recognising how you are feeling and how others around you are feeling. A good way of developing emotional intelligence is to replay past situations in your mind and consider what emotions

people in the situations (including yourself) were experiencing.

Emotional intelligence will enable you to have more control of your emotions, and be able to influence others on an emotional level.

It might also be worth learning more about body language as 80% of communication is non-verbal.

5. Honest Feedback

Honest feedback about yourself is important for self-awareness. Any feedback should come from a person that only wants to help you to improve yourself. If you suspect that feedback coming from a person is because of their own self-interest or because of another agenda, think carefully about its bias.

You can get feedback from family, friends, work colleagues, customers, practically anyone. Usually all you have to do is ask.

It's good to know about the 5 to 1 ratio. The person giving you feedback should give you 5 authentic compliments to 1 piece of specific constructive criticism.

The person you ask for feedback may not have heard of the 5 to 1 ratio. It might be worth discussing it with them prior to asking for feedback. It would also be good if you started using the 5 to 1 ratio when you give feedback to others.

6. List Your Strengths and Weaknesses

Make a list of your strengths and weaknesses. Celebrate your strengths and come up with a plan to develop any areas of weakness.

7. Encourage Open Questions

Encourage open questions that stimulate debate and discussion in all areas of your life. Debating and discussing opinions is a really good way to become more self-aware and develop awareness of others.

8. Know Your Story

The stories we tell ourselves, especially those about ourselves give insight to all things self-awareness. Know your story. Know how your past influences your now and how it could potentially impact on your future. Listen carefully to the narrative.

If their narrative is highly negative or too critical, you may want to sit down and rewrite your story on paper. Once you've done that start telling yourself and others your new story.

9. Life Goals

Write down your life goals. This exercise is brilliant for self-awareness, especially if you practice introspection as you develop your life goals.

10. Coaching

I've never had coaching. But there seems to be a widely held belief that good coaching encourages self-awareness. I can see how this would work. Like most things, the more you put into coaching in terms of self-awareness, the more you'll get out of it.

11. Our Own Version of the Truth

Two people can experience the same event, yet have completely different perspectives and views about it. We all have our own version of the truth. Remember this.

12. Psychometric tests

There are many psychometric tests available, each with its own Pros and Cons. Perhaps the most well-known is the Myers Briggs Type Indicator (MBTI) based on the work of

Carl Jung, a psychoanalyst.

A List of Useful Resources

Books
Here is a list of useful books:

Depressive Illness - The Curse of the Strong
Depressive Illness - The Curse of the Strong is a bestselling book all about depression by Psychiatrist Dr Tim Cantopher. This book is outstanding. Every aspect of the book has been created with a reader who is struggling with depression in mind.

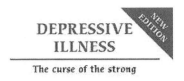

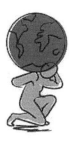

This book is written as if the author is having a conversation with the reader. The book is short, a total of 114 pages, as are the chapters, which is intentional as a symptom of depression is having a limited concentration span. The short chapters mean that the book is easy to dip in and out of. Depressive Illness covers a lot and doesn't waste a single word.

The book covers:

- What depression *really* is and the historic diagnosis and treatment of depression.
- What causes depression.
- What the clinical research around depression says.
- Managing and treatment options for depression.
- Recovery and staying well in the future.
- The politics of depression - why we as a society need to be more open, honest and have dialogue about it.

Cantopher's believes that if you have done too much, been too strong and tried too hard for too long it will lead to clinical depression. This isn't a failing in the person, in fact quite the opposite.

It's a wonder that anyone can be *so* strong for so long. This approach is very empowering for the individual with depression and very true to real life. It is often those that just keep going, those that are there for everyone else who eventually burn out and find themselves in the unpleasant land of clinical depression.

Depressive Illness - The Curse of the Strong is an essential book around clinical depression and should be read by all those interested in mental health and mental illness. For health professionals - particularly in the mental health and illness field this book should be required reading.

The Chimp Paradox – The Mind Management Programme by Dr Steve Peters

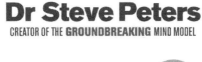

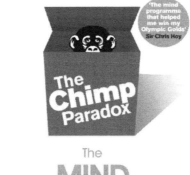

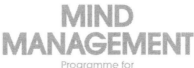

Peters is a Consultant Psychiatrist, who is a Dean for undergraduate students at Sheffield University Medical School. He is also credited with helping athletes achieve success and has worked with: Sky Pro Cycling, Olympic Gold medal winners and Liverpool Football Club.

The Chimp Paradox theory is not a new theory. Peters has taken an old theory and repackaged it, making it more accessible to people. The theory goes that within our mind we have three aspects: the computer, the chimp and the human.

The computer stores autopilots (useful beliefs or behaviours), gremlins (destructive beliefs or behaviours that are removable/changeable in the computer) and goblins (destructive beliefs or behaviours that are difficult to remove/change). All of these are based on past experiences. The computer also holds the values and beliefs that we live our lives by.

The chimp is the emotional part of your brain and is wired for survival and procreation. Whenever the chimp perceives a threat he will decide to fight, flight or freeze. The chimp can hijack you and is responsible for often irrational or destructive behaviours.

The human on the other hand is the logical and rational part of you. The problem comes that the chimp responds 5 times quicker than the human. So it is up to the human to learn to manage the chimp and to change the programming of the computer, so that all parts of the brain work towards the same goals without conflict.

Although this psychological book is not completely focused around mental health, it explains how different parts of the brain work in an easy to understand way. It provides some great strategies for managing life and maintaining good mental health. It also provides some great coping strategies for dealing with pressure, stress and when life doesn't go our way. All of this makes The Chimp Paradox essential reading.

Reasons To Stay Alive by Matt Haig

After reading the unique and brilliant novel The Humans by Matt Haig, I decided to Google this extraordinary Author to learn more about him.

I discovered that he had suffered with poor mental health in the past and was releasing Reasons To Stay Alive, a book on the topic of mental health. So I immediately ordered the book to see what he had to say on the subject.

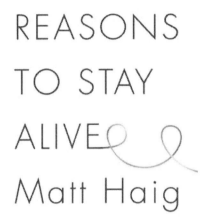

In Reasons To Stay Alive, Haig shares his own experience of anxiety and depression, starting with a note to the reader explaining that these are *his* experiences and that other people might experience anxiety and depression in differing ways. Reasons To Stay Alive was an international bestseller for weeks, perhaps even months.

His book is split into five sections. His first is *Falling* where he writes about symptoms, suicide (including some of the reasons why men are more at risk of suicide) and the facts about depression and anxiety.

Throughout the book there are little gems of good advice.

The second section is *Landing* where he writes a lot about some of his key experiences, as well as the warning signs of depression and anxiety.

The third section is *Rising* where Haig covers panic attacks, the importance of love, how to be there for someone with depression or anxiety and famous people that have suffered from depression and anxiety. This entire section aims to tell someone experiencing poor mental health that they are **not alone**.

Living is the fourth section of the book and focuses on recovery from depression and anxiety. This section covers the importance of slowing down, lists reasons to live, lists things that make Haig's mental health worse and sometimes better.

Being is the last section of the book and gives forty pieces of advice that Haig feels are helpful.

The presentation of the book is good. It's a small white hardback book, with small chapters (some only a page long), his writing style makes it easy-to-read and engaging.

Reasons To Stay Alive is one of the better books written about mental illness on the market. It is well worth a read.

Haig's follow up book, *Notes on a Nervous Planet*, has also become an international bestseller.

Sane New World – Taming the Mind by Ruby Wax

The self-acclaimed poster girl for mental health Ruby Wax went to Oxford University and completed a Masters in Mindfulness-based Cognitive Therapy. Wax wanted to understand the neuroscience behind her own mental health and maybe find a better way to manage her mental health.

On completion of Wax's Masters she wanted to share her own mental health story, along with what she'd learned at Oxford. So she embarked on a tour of mental institutions, before widening the tour to the general public.

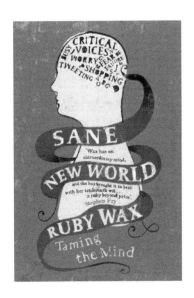

Sane New World is a funny, informative and captivating book on the subject of mental health. It's easily the best book I've ever read on the topic. So it is a *MUST* read for anyone interested in or whom has experienced mental illness.

Sane New World Wax covers:

- What Drives Us Crazy.
- The Critical Inner Voice(s).
- Emotions.
- Depression, Anxiety, OCD, Stress, etc.
- How Our Brain's Work – Neuroscience.
- The Functions of Serotonin, Dopamine, Oxytocin, Cortisol and Other Chemicals in the brain and body.
- How Our Brains Grow and thought/emotional/behavioural patterns can be changed.
- The basics of Mindfulness.
- Some good, but brief mindfulness exercises.
- Alternatives to Mindfulness (if it *isn't your sort of thing* or doesn't work for you).

Throughout the book Wax tells her story. Sane New World includes some wonderful illustrations that give an insight into how Wax operates and is relatable to all. After all, we are all human beings and all being stretched by life to the point of breaking. If we're not careful we might actually break. We need to take hold of the reins in our minds and in our life and if necessary make some changes.

Sane New World will improve your understanding of mental health, teach you how to be and remain mentally and emotionally healthy. It is an enjoyable read. It will teach you how to be in control of your mind, rather than it being in control of you. Definitely worth the investment in my humble opinion.

How To Be Human – The Manual by Ruby Wax

How To Be Human is insightful, funny, warm and engaging. A pleasure to read. It's like somebody is pouring wisdom into your head while you're having a chat with them.

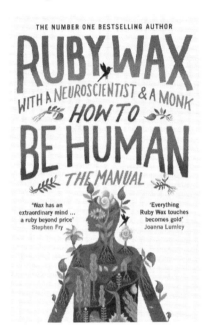

Each chapter covers a topic and is wittily written by Wax. For each chapter Wax has consulted with Ash Ranpura, a Neuroscientist and Gelong Thubten, a Buddhist Monk.

At the end of each chapter are fascinating transcripts of these discussions.

Interspersed throughout How To Be Human, Wax shares some of her own mental illness story.

So what exactly does Wax cover in How To Be Human? Pretty much everything. Here is the title of each chapter:

- Evolution
- Thoughts
- Emotions
- The Body
- Compassion
- Relationships
- Sex
- Kids
- Addiction
- The Future
- Mindfulness Exercises
- Forgiveness

How To Be Human builds on the strong foundations of Wax's two previously published books: Sane New World – Taming the Mind and A Mindfulness Guide for the Frazzled.

A Mindfulness Guide for the Frazzled by Ruby Wax

A Mindfulness Guide for the Frazzled is split into sections, which include: an introduction to Mindfulness, Neuroscience and How Our Brains Work, a six-week Mindfulness Course, Mindfulness for Parents, Babies & Children, Mindfulness for Older Kids & Teenagers and Mindfulness & Wax.

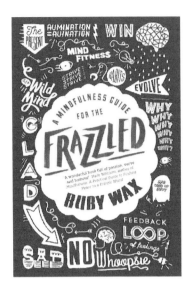

Wax's story sections spattered throughout Frazzled were fascinating to read. Wax's occasional drawings and photos throughout the book were also enjoyable.

It was interesting to see the two MRI brain scans on Wax in Frazzled. One was taken before a week-long silence mindfulness meditative retreat and one afterwards.

The format and structure of Frazzled is pleasing, although Wax could have added a section on Mindfulness for older people.

The six-week Mindfulness Course pages are grey-edged, which makes it easy for the reader to find the course. The exercises in the course did feel repetitive to read and it felt like whole sections from Week 1 had been copy/pasted into the other weeks of the course.

Frazzled shouldn't be compared with Sane New World but it's difficult not to compare the two books. Frazzled is just as informative as *Sane New World* but not as funny. *Frazzled* reads like a self-help instructional book on Mindfulness. This is great if mindfulness is for you, but not everyone is as into mindfulness as Wax is.

Useful Websites
Useful Websites include:

1. NHS Choices is crammed with health information. Information on health conditions, treatments, medications, public health issues, carers rights, services, practically everything you could ever want to know about health and healthcare in the UK. Delivered by the NHS you can be assured that the information is correct, up to date and based on research and evidence.

It has some great online tools such as: BMI Calculator, Mood self-assessment, Sleep self-assessment and many more.

2. Mind's website is a treasure trove of mental health and mental illness information. It has an A-Z listing of mental health conditions, information about treatments, advice on how to support someone with mental illness, legal advice, urgent help advice and stories of people with mental illness.

3. CALM (Campaign Against Living Miserably) is a movement against male suicide.

CALM offers support for men who are feeling low or in crisis. They campaign for a change in culture, encouraging men to talk about how they are feeling and aim to eliminate the stigma of men seeking help due to mental illness. They hope to prevent as many male suicides as possible and also offer support for those affected by suicide.

4. SANE is a mental health charity credited with the Black Dog Campaign and the #EndTheStigma hashtag. The phrase *black dog* comes from Winston Churchill who described his depression as a *black dog*. SANE has also worked with Ruby Wax who coined the term *Black Dog Tribe*.

5. Rethink Mental Illness is a mental health charity that have a vast amount of information about mental health and mental illness on their website. Rethink also deliver a wide range of services and support including: support groups, helplines, advocacy and information about housing, criminal justice and employment.

6. Patient.info has a A-Z list of articles written by doctors, information videos, a symptom checker and an active online community. On more than one occasion while at work in the NHS, I've seen doctors checking this valuable website.

7. NetDoctor is similar to Patient.Info, but with more of a focus on healthy living and healthy eating.

8. Head Meds tells you everything you ever wanted to know about medications for mental illnesses. It also gives information about conditions and shares people stories of mental illness. What I particularly like about this website is that it tells you how the medications affect sex, alcohol, weight, sleep and just about everything else.

A useful website that I always visit before medication reviews or at times when there's discussions about changing my medication.

9. eMC (Medicines.org.uk) is a useful website for looking up information about medicines.

I use <u>British National Formulary (BNF)</u> but the medical terminology can be difficult for someone from a non-medical or non-nursing background to understand. This is why eMC made it on this list instead of the BNF.

10. <u>Bipolar UK</u> has a great online eCommunity. I use it all the time and find it a very useful resource. People on the eCommunity are friendly and share their experiences around a wide range of topics.

The eCommunity goes a long way to making you feel less isolated by reassuring you that you're not the only one experiencing what you are. They also have support groups that are run by volunteers who are people living with bipolar. I used to go to a local group before it shut down and found it invaluable on my road to recovery.

11. The <u>Samaritans</u> offer support by telephone, in person, email or by writing. Their telephone number and email are open 24/7/365, being a lifeline to people in a mental illness crisis.

12. <u>Time To Change</u> aims to end mental health discrimination. They do so by education in schools and by supporting employers. They have a wealth of information online including myths/facts, conditions, how to support your friend and a quiz to test your knowledge on mental health.

13. The <u>Mental Health Foundation's </u>website has some informative publications which you can download or order a printed copy. Their *vision* is for everyone in the UK to have good mental health.

14. <u>Anxiety UK</u> has been around since the 70s and provides a wide range resources around anxiety. Its website is informative, they offer an info line, a text service and training to

organisations and companies.

15. <u>Office of National Statistics – Health and Social Care</u> is the best place to find statistical information about health. It is regularly updated based on data from the NHS, Local Authories and other Government Departments in the UK.

16. <u>National Institute of Clinical Excellence (NICE)</u> provides pathways, guidelines and advice across the UK for the best possible evidence-based healthcare. The guidance they provide is developed by groups of clinical experts who provide experience of what works in practice and by examining and analysing research.

If you want to know what care you or a relative or friend should be receiving and check that it's of a high quality then visit NICE's website.

17. <u>Health For Teens</u> I found while doing research for this chapter. It's specifically aimed at teenagers and looks appealing. They even create content in consultation with young people. I think the name of the website maybe off-putting to young people though – but this is just my personal opinion.

Part 2 - Empathy Through Lived Experience

I've Been One of the 1 in 4

At any one time, 1 in 4 people are experiencing poor mental health, albeit to varying degrees of severity.

I have experienced poor mental health at different times in my life and to varying degrees, as have many other people I know.

Depending on what I'm thinking and how I'm feeling, I've used a number of strategies to manage my own mental and emotional health, including:

- Reminding myself that my mental or emotional state is temporary and will change.
- Monitoring my mind and mood to look for improvement or deterioration.
- Keeping my negative internal voice in check.
- Asking for help, support and understanding from family & friends.
- Off-loading to friends.
- Distraction.
- Sleeping.
- Taking time out to rest and relax.
- Meditating.
- Imagining and Visualising a better future – giving me hope that things will get better.
- Reading for pleasure.
- Having an up-beat music playlist.
- Being creative to connect with and nourish my soul.
- Visiting my GP.

The Death of Robin Williams

In 2014, the death of Robin Williams, the Actor & Comedian by suicide shocked and saddened me. Robin had suffered with severe clinical depression.

We should talk about mental health. We should know how to look after our own mental health and how to best support our loved ones that are experiencing poor mental health. Too many people die because of their poor mental health. Robin Williams was one of these too many people.

**The Impact of Mental Illness on the Individual, Family &
Friends**

Mental illness can have a massive impact on the individual.
As well as the symptoms of the particular mental illness, they
can also experience:

- A decreased quality of life. Worse physical health with
  an increase in bacterial and viral infections due
  having a weakened immune response.
- Issues with self-esteem or confidence - This goes hand
  in hand with the symptoms of mental illness.
- Fear of judgement or being stigmatised - This comes
  from societal and cultural attitudes to mental illness.
- Discrimination - People may treat them differently or
  worst once people know about their mental illness.
- Education or training difficulties - They may struggle
  to complete education or training, particularly if they
  are unwell. This can lead to problems with
  employment opportunities.
- Employment - They may have problems getting or
  maintaining a job. This might be due to the number of
  sick days they have if their mental illness is unstable.
- Poverty - They are more likely to earn less which puts
  them at higher risk of living in poverty, with all the
  additional challenges and stress that this brings.
- Financial - They may have problems with debt due to
  over spending when unwell or through just finding it
  too difficult to survive on a low income.
- Romantic relationship breakdown - This might be due
  to money problems mentioned above, or due to the
  fact that they have little or no interest in sex (a very

common symptom of a mental illness), or because of both.

- Breakdown in other meaningful relationships - This maybe caused things people say or do when mentally ill. Or it may be caused by the person with mental illness deliberately choosing to isolate themselves.
- Legal issues - They may commit criminal activity and have contact with the Police or Probation Service. In Prisons the percentage of people that have mental illness is much higher than that in the general population. This suggests that people with mental illness are either more likely to be involved in crime or that society sometimes treats mental illness as a criminal justice issue, rather than a health issue.

Family & Friends

The family and friends of an individual with mental illness can have a tough time. But it can also be rewarding to. They can experience:

- Breakdown in relationship with the individual with mental illness due to the person being seen as unreliable, unpredictable and sometimes even as unsupportive.
- A *possible* decreased quality of life. This is possible for family or friends that spend all of the time looking after someone with a mental illness. Family and friends have a right to their own full lives as well.
- Fear of getting the same mental illness - This is usually in siblings or children.
- A wide range of emotions including: guilt, anger, shame, embarrassment, jealousy, resentment,

frustration, confusion, compassion, understanding, empathy, denial and a feeling of relief. These emotions come at different times. If someone is struggling with particularly negative or difficult emotions, it might be worth them speaking to their General Practitioner (GP) about counselling.

- Caring responsibilities - Family and friends might need to care for the person with mental illness. This care could range from occasional help to daily assistance. This care could include: personal care, monitoring their thoughts, emotions and behaviours, managing medication and financial support.
- Financial Pressure - This might come from the costs associated with caring for person with mental illness, reduced income through only working part time to care for the person with mental illness or trying to bail them out of debt.
- Poverty - With all the additional challenges and stress that this brings.
- Worrying about the future of the person with mental illness. Or the opposite, not worrying about the individual's future as they manage their own illness well with good support networks and good coping strategies.
- Stress or chronic stress - caused by caring responsibilities.
- Feeling that the support services are not giving enough support to the individual with mental illness or their family & friends.
- Breakdown in romantic relationships or other meaningful relationships as all the attention, energy

and money is being used to support the person with the mental illness.

The impact of mental illness on the individual, family and friends can be significant. But there are ways to manage illnesses and cope with the challenges.

The End of the World

Catastrophic thinking is imagining the worst possible outcome of future events. It could be an upcoming social event, a meeting at work, anything really. Big or small events. Your mind whirls with all the possibilities of everything going completely wrong. You might start to get a feeling of dread in the pit of your stomach. Ultimately you think that it's the end of the world.

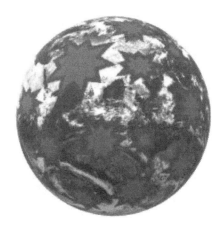

This way of thinking is totally unbalanced, is unhelpful and is ultimately driven by anxiety and fear. If you look back after the event, you'll probably find that none of what you imagined ever took place. And even if the worst did happen, you'll discover that you dealt with it just fine.

We've all had times when catastrophic thinking takes over our mind, were our bodies pumps out sweat and we may have even started to shake. We need to be aware of catastrophic thinking and challenge it early on, before it gets out of hand and leaves us paralysed.

Start by gathering evidence that contradicts your thoughts. These might be things like finding out what the meeting at work is about beforehand, meaning our thoughts can't make up all sorts of nightmare scenarios about us being rubbish at our job and that it is a meeting about performance. Another example, if your thoughts are telling you that someone hates you, go talk to the person. Ask them what they think of you. There's no stronger evidence that getting information direct from the source.

Next remember all the times your catastrophic thinking has been wrong. All the possibilities that were imagined but never happened. Now reassure your mind by thinking: *Nothing is ever as bad as I think it will be. These thoughts come from anxiety. I can handle whatever happens at this event.* Repeat this phrase a few times if you are still struggling.

Now think about and focus on how well the future event could go. Imagine all the positive possibilities. If there's anything you can prepare or do to make the event more likely to go well, do it. Doing a task will also serve as a distraction from your thoughts. If there's nothing you can prepare or do, but you still want to do something to distract you from your thoughts, see Part 3 - Life Hacks, A List of Distraction Activities chapter of this book.

Take a deep breath in, hold it for 15 seconds, then breath out. Taking a moment to breathe gives you an opportunity to be present in the moment and can help lessen the intensity of catastrophic thinking.

After the event take time to reflect. Think about the event and how none of the devastation you imagined happened. Use this as a tool for the future. So next time you begin to think the worst for a future event, remind yourself that it won't be as bad as what you think. In fact, it could be the opposite of what you think and be a really positive experience.

A final idea: Think about sharing your thoughts, feelings, behaviours and reflections with someone you can trust. It can be really good to use someone as a sounding board to get an overview of any situation. If they were at or involved with the event, even better. They can share what they thought and felt. They can also give you some honest feedback about your behaviour and whether your thoughts beforehand were justified or not.

Catastrophic thinking can never be justified because the thoughts com from anxiety and anxiety isn't rational.

Rumination & Critical Inner Voice

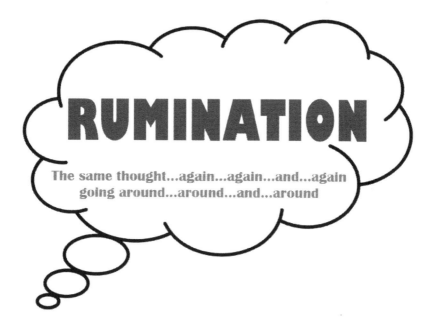

Rumination is thinking the same thoughts or replaying memories again, again and again in your mind. Nothing good ever comes from it. It's like having a song that you hate on full ear-bleeding volume and stuck on repeat. Rumination makes you feel like you are losing your mind.

When it comes to replaying memories, they are usually memories that are emotionally traumatic. Our memory of events is never accurate and always has a negative bias. What you need to remember if you find yourself ruminating is that the event has happened. It's in the past. It's gone. You can't change what's happened, no matter how many times you replay the video. It's time to accept what's happened, how it made you feel, so that you can let it go and move on.

Rumination is a waste of time, energy and effort. Rumination and the Critical Inner Voice go together. The critical inner voice is that voice inside your head that says things like:

- You're not good enough.
- You don't know what you're doing.
- Just *who* do you think you are?
- You're worthless.
- You screw everything up. You are a screw up.
- Nobody cares about you.

The critical inner voice is abusive and says things that you wouldn't dream of saying to your worst enemy. It never says anything useful, nice, good or kind. It tends to get louder and louder if we allow it to. Managing the critical inner voice starts with the choice not to put up with the things it says to you.

I manage my critical inner voice in two main ways. First by imagining a volume control knob. I imagine it being turned down and hear the voice go quieter and quieter until it is silent. Second, I repeat positive affirmations that I know are true. I say things to myself like:

- I am good at my job. I have a lot of specialist knowledge and thirteen years of clinical experience.
- I offer a lot to people around me, including humour, compassion and kindness.
- People value my opinion. I know this because I am often asked for it by others.
- I am doing the best that I can and learn every day.

Having difficulty coming up with positive affirmations about yourself that are true? Ask people who are close to you: What is positive about me? What do you like about me? Others often see things that we don't spot in ourselves.

Transactional Analysis: One Way to Influence Others

Dr Eric Berne developed a brilliant theory on transactional analysis. It has three roles: the parent, the adult and the child. I've used this theory countless times to influence others and manage social interactions.

It has been so helpful in my life, that I feel it should be taught to everyone.

Parent

In any interaction with others every person takes on one of the three roles. The parent can be either nurturing or critical. The nurturing parent comes from a place of compassion and care for the other person or people.

The other person or people are usually in the child role. The parent role has many drawbacks, which can include taking on all of the work in a task. They will act as mother hen and will use phrases like:

- Everything will be okay.
- I'll do...to solve your problem.
- Are you okay if I do...
- I'll take care of you.

The critical parent is harsh to the other person or people who are usually in the child role. They will look for mistakes or problems and act in domineering or authoritarian way. One of the drawbacks, is that they can be demotivating to others by being overly critical. They will use phrases like:

- Don't do it *that* way, do it this way...
- You haven't thought about...

- You need to do...
- Why haven't you done it in the *right* way?

Adult

The adult is seen as the most useful and ideal for any interaction. The best outcomes in social interactions are achieved when both parties are in the adult role. The adult role is one that comes from a place of reason, logic and assertiveness. The adult actively listens and doesn't let their emotions govern them or the social interaction. The adult role is thought to be the most balanced of the roles. They will use phrases like:

- How can we work together to achieve our shared goal?
- Tell me more about...
- What are the barriers? What do we need to overcome the barriers?
- I *think* you should do that as I am already doing this. That would be an equally shared distribution of work.

Child

The child role has two aspects: the curious child and the adaptive child. The child role comes from a place of emotions. The curious child is interested in learning, creativity and possibilities. They are usually driven by intrigue, interest and excitement.

The adaptive child reacts to the situation either by changing themselves to fit in with the situation or rebelling (this usually causing conflict in the social situation).

The other person or people are usually in the parent role.

The other person or people are usually in the parent role. The child role has many draw backs which can include not being interested in the detailed tasks that need to be completed in order to achieve shared goals or taking no responsibility for their actions. They will use phrases like:

- I want to learn more about...
- I think a novel solution to the problem could be...
- I could do this or take on this role...
- I hate that idea. I don't want to do that at all.

During a social interaction, the other person or people will either go to the opposite role to yours or match your role. Which happens depends on the individuals and the social situation.

Possible Combinations of Parent, Adult and Child Roles

There are 9 possible combinations using the transactional analysis theory:

Transactional Analysis

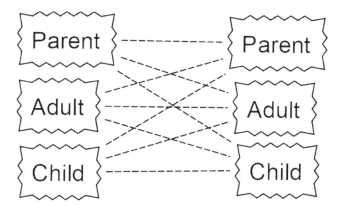

by Dr Eric Berne

Parent and Parent - This is a difficult mode for two people to work in, as they both want to be in control, make the decisions and want others to follow their lead.

Parent and Adult - This can be a productive mode if the person in the adult role is willing to take the lead of the person in the parent role. The person in the parent role also needs to have a balanced approach. The difficulties with this combination often come from the person in the parent role being overly nurturing or overly critical.

Parent and Child - This combination usually results in the person in the parent role doing all the work. This can lead to feelings of resentment during or after the social interaction.

Adult and Parent - This dynamic causes tension as the person in the adult role can feel the person in the parent role is being condescending. The person in the adult role can also feel frustrated by the language the person in the parent role uses.

Adult and Adult - This is generally the most ideal way for two people to interact socially, in sharing of work and achieving shared goals.

Adult and Child - This combination can be effective for working together, as long as both are happy in their roles and share the work evenly. For the person in the child role, it can really help them in they are prone to procrastination, as they know that they'll have to answer to the person in the adult role. Although this is a great dynamic for work-based relationships where you have a manager and an employee, it isn't so great for personal relationships.

Child and Parent - This combination leads to the person in the role of the parent usually getting very frustrated with the person in the role of a child.

Child and Adult - This dynamic leads to the person in the role of the adult usually getting very frustrated with the person in the role of a child.

Child and Child - People in these roles often have a great time together, with lots of fun. But they struggle to get any work or anything productive done.

How to Use the Theory
To use this theory, you need to be self-aware enough to recognise which role you and others are in (parent, adult or child).

Once you have this information, you can make a conscious

decision to switch your role. Usually when you consciously switch your role, the other person or people will unconscious switch their role to the opposite role to yours or the same role depending on the individual or situation.

It's useful to know that certain people or social settings can make us automatically go into a role. For example, I used to have a departmental manager than would make me slip into the role of the child every time I interacted with her.

Once I recognised that the departmental manager used to make me slip into the role of the child, during a social interaction I consciously switched my role to that of the Adult. The departmental manager switched their role without even realising, hovering between Parent and Adult.

Severe Clinical Depression?

In January 2015, everything stopped. I stopped being able to function and was ill.

The truth is that I had been ill for a long time before this, but that I had continued to solider on – hoping that I would start to feel better.

Here were some of my symptoms:

☑ No concentration span. I wasn't able to watch TV or films, read or write. I didn't feel safe to drive, so I didn't.

☑ Short-term memory loss.

☑ Feeling constantly exhausted despite sleeping for many, many hours.

☑ Some insomnia and night terrors.

☑ Back pain – despite resting and regularly completing physiotherapy exercises.

☑ Headaches.

☑ Stomach ache/constipation despite eating a reasonably good diet.

☑ Poor personal hygiene and not cleaning my home environment.

☑ Overeating or forcing myself to eat despite feeling that I didn't want to.

☑ No motivation – I found it extremely difficult and tiring to do the smallest of tasks.

☑ Reckless spending of money – mostly through online shopping.

☑ Any extremely variable mood which changed throughout the day and night. From being void of any feelings to a tornado of fast swirling feelings including: guilt, inadequacy and feeling like a failure.

☑Anxiety – resulting in becoming antisocial and finding it difficult to leave home.

☑Worry and panic about what people would think of me.

☑Feeling hopeless, which is the worst feeling in the world.

☑Feeling like I was losing my mind.

☑Feeling like I was falling down a dark bottomless pit.

☑Feeling frustrated at not being able to *snap out of it* and that nothing I did made a difference to how I felt or my ability to function.

☑Overly self-critical thoughts and zero self-esteem.

☑A critical inner voice that was loud and repetitive.

☑At two particularly bad points I suffered from compulsions to end my life.

☑In short, feeling like my mind, body and soul were being devoured and destroyed by this illness.

So I went to see my GP who completed the PHQ depression test and diagnosed me with **severe clinical depression**. At several points throughout my treatment, this test was repeated to check on my progress. At one point, I was scoring 24 out of a possible 27. My GP started me on antidepressants and encouraged me to self-refer for counselling.

The first antidepressant didn't work, despite gradually increasing the dose to the maximum. This is really common, happening to at least 50% of people. So my GP gradually withdrew the first antidepressant and then started me on another – which thankfully started working. I self-referred to counselling, had an assessment and after a short time on the waiting list, began therapy sessions.

January to May 2015 felt like a *write-off* in every sense of the word. I felt extremely lucky to have made it through this dark and difficult time.

Looking back, I'd had depressive tendencies for at least the last few years before getting really ill. I'd been rubbish at spotting the symptoms in myself, but have come out of the experience much more aware of signs, symptoms and triggers now.

By May 2015, I felt in recovery. I was still on the antidepressants and I'd started taking multivitamins to make sure my body and mind was getting what it needed to function. I felt good, better than I had in years. I'd even started laughing again, proper belly laughs, which I hadn't done for what felt like forever.

I thanked those close to me for their support, love, care and kindness. But then things started to get worse...

My Life Hiatus – Inpatient Admission

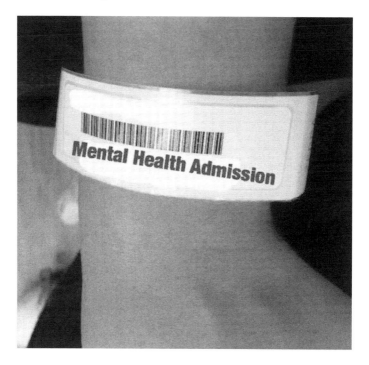

In September 2015, I had to take an unexpected what-I-call *Life Hiatus*. My mental health had gradually deteriorated to the point where I was having severe and erratic mood swings. Everyone's mood fluctuates throughout the day, but not to the extremes I was experiencing.

People talk about good and bad days with depression. I was having good, bad, okay or mixed mood states lasting between 45 minutes to 4-6 hours. These mood swings were unpredictable with no pattern. They didn't have triggers and were not related to my critical inner voice.

These mood swings were torturous. See *My Mood Swing Table* in the next chapter for details of what these mood swings were like.

I felt desperate for the mood swings to end. To the point of having suicidal ideation and a clear plan of action.

I had thought that I was objective about my mental health. But because the mood swings had gradually got worse, I hadn't realised how unwell I was. I sought help because three people close to me said that I wasn't well. Luckily, I had these people around me and I knew that could trust them, even if I couldn't trust myself.

So I went to my local A&E. I was assessed by a Mental Health Nurse and together we decided that I needed admission. I stayed on the A&E Ward overnight, whilst I waited for an available bed on a mental health ward.

The next evening, I was transferred to a mental health ward. On arrival at the ward, my possessions were searched and Nursing Staff took my shoe laces, belt, hoodie (due to cord in hood), phone charger, lighters and medication. The ward layout was a square shaped main corridor with dormitories, individual rooms and many other rooms that where behind locked doors.

The first night was terrifying. Everything about the place was frightening. The environment. The locked doors. The routine. The rules I hadn't been told. The other patients. The staff. At one point, I was physically shaking in terror.

I was assessed by a Psychiatrist and commenced on 10-minute observations. It would be a few days before I was reviewed. At the time, I couldn't understand why they appeared to be doing very little to help me and my state of mind. But afterwards, I realised that they had wanted to observe me and see my mood swings for themselves.

The Consultant Psychiatrist diagnosed me with cyclothymic disorder (a form of Bipolar). This diagnosis means lifelong mood stabiliser and/or antidepressant medication, but I didn't realise this at the time and nobody told me.

The Consultant Psychiatrist informed me that they were reluctant to give any other diagnosis on a person's first admission to a mental health ward. I told the Consultant Psychiatrist that I didn't care what she wanted to called it, as long as they gave me some medication that worked. I explained that with some stability in mood, I could make further psychological and behavioural changes to help myself to get well.

I was started on Quetiapine, an antipsychotic and mood stabilising medication. It was to help to take the edge off my mood swings and give me some stability of mood. I was also started on Mirtazapine, an antidepressant. This was to help to manage the depression/low moods.

Overall, I was an in-patient on the mental health ward for about 12 days. During this time, my Mum and good friend Steve were superb. They took over all my responsibilities and made sure that everything in the outside world was sorted, meaning that I didn't have to worry about anything – apart from getting better.

I will never be able to thank Mum and Steve enough for what they did for me, but I have repeatedly thanked them anyway. I will never be able to explain how much I appreciate everything that they did for me.

I feel that I got to this crisis point because I waited so long to get referred to and assessed by Community Mental Health Services.

It feels like Community Mental Health Services are designed to keep people out, rather than let people in. This is probably due to of a lack of resources. But it really doesn't help to support people with mental illnesses to get and stay well.

I was discharged from the hospital and engaged with Community Mental Health Services. I recognised that Recovery would be a slow and progressive one.

My Mood Swing Table

Highs:

- *Physical Symptoms:* High energy levels. Very productive. Difficulty in getting/staying asleep. Headaches. Speaking Quickly. Hypersexualised.

- *Mental / Cognitive Symptoms:* Racing thoughts – lots of ideas, but struggling to focus on one for long enough. Difficulty in concentrating. A rush of ideas for creative projects. Saying whatever I think without considering the implications of what I'm saying. Grandiose thinking – Thinking I can do anything to a level beyond the level of an expert. Thinking that I understand things on a much deeper level than everyone else. Short-term memory loss. Insomnia and night terrors.

- *Emotional Symptoms:* Excessively joyful with no reason for this state of mood. Super confident. Loads of self-esteem. Excessively excited again without reason. Feeling like I can do anything. Feeling frustrated or irritable without a reason. Varying levels of anxiety, from worried to outright panic.

- *Behavioural Examples:* Being super productive. Being overtly social. Take on too many commitments, thinking that I can do everything. Impulsive behaviours – including excessive shopping, even when I don't have the money. Unfinished tasks – sometimes being unable to focus for long enough on tasks to complete them.

Okays:

- *Physical Symptoms:* Relatively symptom free. Considering the extreme High and Low physical symptoms.

- *Mental / Cognitive Symptoms:* Slower mental and cognitive functioning, compared to when I was well.

- *Emotional Symptoms:* Void of any emotion. Zombified. Feeling like what I imagine a zombie feels like. Going through the motions.

- *Behavioural Examples:* Able to function, but only *just.*

Lows:

- *Physical Symptoms:* Exhaustion – despite sleeping for many, many hours. Back pain and stomach pain that doesn't resolve with appropriate treatments. Headaches. Constipation. Physical anxiety symptoms: raised pulse and blood pressure.

- *Mental / Cognitive Symptoms:* Limited/no concentration span. Short-term memory loss. Critical inner voice. Negative thoughts about what other people think about me. Insomnia and night terrors. Concern about losing my mind.

- *Emotional Symptoms:* Despair and hopelessness. No confidence and rock bottom self-esteem. Feeling frustrated or irritable without a reason. Feeling like I am falling down a dark bottomless pit. Feeling guilt, inadequacy and feeling like a failure. Varying levels of anxiety, from worried to outright panic. Desperation – wanting the mental and emotional anguish to end. Feeling like my mind, body and soul are being devoured and destroyed.

- *Behavioural Examples:* Loss of interest in leisure activities. Unable to watch TV, read or do other leisure activities. Overeating or forcing myself to eat despite having no appetite. Poor personal hygiene. No motivation. Reckless spending of money – mostly through online shopping to make myself feel temporarily better. Social anxiety – isolating myself and avoiding social situations.

Mixed Mood States:

- *Physical Symptoms:* A mix of high, low and okay physical symptoms to varying degrees of severity.

- *Mental / Cognitive Symptoms:* A mix of high, low and okay mental / cognitive symptoms to varying degrees of severity. Concern about losing my mind. Concern about what mood would come next and its severity.

- *Emotional Symptoms:* A mix of high, low and okay emotional symptoms to varying degrees of severity.

- *Behavioural Examples:* A mix of high, low and okay behaviours to varying degrees of severity.

Signs that Someone is Struggling

Spotting the signs that someone is struggling with mental illness is really important, especially because they might not realise that they are struggling themselves.

Here are some of the signs, looking back on my own experiences, that I was struggling. These can be applied to anyone:

- Changes in social contact. Usually they are less social than normal, withdrawn and opting to isolate themselves from others. This may include: making excuses for not going to social events and arriving late and leaving early at social events. For some mental health illnesses, such as mania in bipolar they may be more social.
- Changes in their environment. There's usually more mess, a build up of used plates & cutlery, over flowing bins, basically chaos.
- Changes to their appearance. They make less effort with their appearance, hair might be dishevelled, clothes might not be ironed, the same clothes worn for days, weight loss or gain and potentially body odour.
- Changes in expression of emotion. They may be emotionally closed, displaying none of their feelings. Or expression of emotions might be overt. Sadness and crying or easily frustrated and quick to anger.
- Over thinking and over analysing things.
- Smoking more. Increased alcohol and/or drug use.
- Loss of ambitions and dreams.
- Be having difficulties in work or off work due to sickness.

- Having no future plans.
- Changes to sleeping pattern. They may sleep more or less, suffer with insomnia or wake up every day exhausted. They will usually report having less energy.
- Saying bizarre things.
- Talking about suicide or ending their life. They may express a strong desire for everything to be over.
- Being overly self-critical.
- Seemingly to lack care about anyone or anything.
- Not actively listening to others or being able to retain information given.

If you see these signs in family members or friends, it might be worth having an honest, yet sensitive, conversation with them about what you've noticed. It might be worth encouraging them to go and speak to their GP.

You can find out more about supporting someone with Mental Illness in Part 3 - Life Hacks section of this book, in the chapter titled How to Support Someone with Mental Illness.

My Mental Health & Illness Playlist

Music can have a huge influence on mental health. That written, music isn't a cure for mental illness. If you want to find a 'cure' read the Treatments & Recovery chapter in Part 1 of this book.

Here is my playlist of brilliant songs that I associate with mental health & illness:

Under Pressure - **Queen**

I Miss You - **Blink-182**

A Change of Heart - **The 1975**

Obsessions - **Marina And The Diamonds**

Don't Look Back In Anger - **OASIS**

True Colors - **Eva Cassidy**

Thank You - **Alanis Morissette**

Lights - **Ellie Goulding**

Heart Out - **The 1975**

7 Minutes In Heaven - **Fall Out Boy**

Wake Me Up When September Ends - **Green Day**

Message In A Bottle - **The Police**

Don't Rain On My Parade - **Barbara Streisand**

Favorite Scars - **Cher**

Kids In The Dark - **All Time Low**

Get Here - **Oleta Adams**

Things Will Go My Way (Acoustic) - **The Calling**

Make You Feel My Love - **Adelle**

Beautiful - **Christina Aguilera**

Whataya Want From Me - **Adam Lambert**

It's Not Living (If It's Not With You) - **The 1975**

Walking Away - **Craig David**

Born To Try - **Delta Goodrem**

What Do I Know? - **Ed Sheeran**

I'm Still Standing - **Elton John**

Adam's Song - **Blink-182**

Thanks For The Memories - **Fall Out Boy**

Strong Enough - **Cher**

Big Girls Don't Cry - **Fergie**

Fight Song - **Rachel Platten**

Our Lives - **The Calling**

Save Myself - **Ed Sheeran**

I'll Be Okay - **McFly**

How To Save A Life - **The Fray**

I Did It For Everyone - **The Feeling**

Never Let Go - **Bryan Adams**

Nails For Breakfast, Tacks For Snacks - **Panic! At The Disco**

Don't Let The Sun Go Down On Me - **George Michael & Elton John**

A World To Believe In - **Celine Dion**

Help! - **The Beatles**

Vulnerable - **Pet Shop Boys**

We Are Golden - **Mika**

Where We Go - **Pink**

You're A Superstar - **Love Inc.**

Impossible Year - **Panic! At The Disco**

What Doesn't Kill You Makes You Stronger - **Kelly Clarkson**

What Have You Done Today To Make Yourself Feel Proud - **M People**

I Bruise Easily - **Natasha Bedingfield**

Inside Out (Feat. Charlee) - **The Chainsmokers**

Happy Pill - **Troye Sivan**

Try - **Nelly Furtado**

Just Like A Pill - **Pink**

Circle The Drain - **Katy Perry**

Life Is Life - **Noah And The Whale**

Moodswings - **Charlotte Church**

Sunrise - **Norah Jones**

Human - **One Republic**

Run For Your Life - **Matt Cardle**

Soaked - **Adam Lambert**

Everybody Knows - **Leonard Cohen**

Flaws - **Olly Murs**

Life Is A Rollercoaster - **Ronan Keating**

Sensitive Guy - **McBusted**

Morning Sun - **Robbie Williams**

Only A Human - **George Ezra**

Don't Stop Me Now - **Queen**

The Blackest Day - **Lana Del Rey**

I Always Wanna Die (Sometimes) - **The 1975**

Creep - **Radiohead**

Come Undone - **Robbie Williams**

Jealousy - **Will Young**

Happy Ending - **Mika**

Affirmation - **Savage Garden**

Self Control - **Scissor Sisters**

What Do You Take Me For (Ft. Pusha T) - **Pixie Lott**

Mirrors - **Sally Oldfield**

I Want To Break Free - **Queen**

I Don't Feel Like Dancin' - **Scissor Sisters**

Imagine - **John Lennon**

Joy - **Will Young**

Every Traveled Road - **Scott Matthew**

I Can Make You Feel Good - **Shalamar**

Stronger - **Britney Spears**

Crash and Burn - **Savage Garden**

I'm Not Dead - **Pink**

Everything - **Alanis Morissette**

Hold On - **Shawn Mendes**

Not Alone - **McFly**

In My Secret Life - **Leonard Cohen**

This Is My Life - **Shirley Bassey**

Run - **Snow Patrol**

Life Is Worth Living - **Justin Bieber**

Self Inflicted - **Katy Perry**

Up! - **Shania Twain**

The Best - **Tina Turner**

Born This Way - **Lady Gaga**

Stay With Me - **Sam Smith**

I'll Be Your Strength - **The Wanted**

Everybody's Changing - **Keane**

21st Century Life - **Sam Sparro**

Desire - **Years & Years**

I know it's the most eclectic list of songs spanning a wide range of genres. But each to his own.

A good friend of mine has an 'upbeat' music playlist for when he needs motivation. I've ~~stolen~~ creatively imitated his idea. I always have an upbeat album playing in the mornings while I drink my coffee. Coffee and an upbeat album have become my morning essentials for motivation. Give it a try.

The Different Roles within the Mental Health Team

There are a range of different roles within the Mental Health Team. Here is an explanation of each role, in alphabetical order:

Most mental health wards have **Activity Coordinators**. Their job is to organise recreational and potentially therapeutic activities to prevent boredom and break up the monotony of the day. These scheduled activities also help to give a sense of routine and normality.

Art Therapists help patients with mental illness to express their thoughts and feelings through a wide range of art mediums. Mediums could include things like drawing, painting and sculpting clay.

The **Associate Nurses** is a new role to bridge the gap in skills between a registered Nurse and a Support Workers.

As this role is relatively new, it is unclear what role they will play in the Mental Health Team. The role requires registration with the Nursing & Midwifery Council (UK) and the Standard of Proficiency include promoting health, preventing ill health and providing and monitoring care.

It is likely that the Associate Nurse will do prevention of mental illness and promotion of good mental health work. Have contact with patients to monitor their mental illness and reporting of any deterioration to the multi-disciplinary team.

A **Cognitive Behaviour Therapy (CBT) Therapists** will deliver CBT sessions to patients with mental illnesses. You can find out more about CBT in Part 1 - Treatments and

Recovery chapter in section 1 of this book.

Community Psychiatric Nurses (CPNs) play a vital role within the Mental Health Team. They usually have a caseload of patients with mental illnesses. Their role includes: assessments, development of care plans, delivery of psychological or psychosocial interventions (talking therapies), liaising with other members of the multi-disciplinary team, liaison with external services (such as housing, police, probation, GPs, etc.) and reviewing care plans.

Dual Diagnosis Nurses / Practitioners are specialists in working with patients with mental illnesses and other diagnoses. Today these roles are usually for highly complex patients that have a mental illness as well as a learning disability.

There are a high number of patients that have a mental illness and an addiction to and dependency on alcohol or drugs struggle to get support from Mental Health Teams. Often Mental Health Teams will tell patients that the patient needs to address their addiction first. They will then refer patients to community Addiction Services.

Evidence suggests that collaborative working between Mental Health Teams and Addiction Services has the best outcomes. Dual Diagnosis Nurses / Practitioners working between Mental Health Teams and Addiction Services would certainly improve outcomes for this complex patient group.

Family Therapists may be a therapist employed to do specific family work or another therapist that does family therapy as part of their role. The aims of family therapy are to: improve communication between family members, to improve relationships between family members, to help family members deal with conflict and emotions within a safe environment, to help families to deal with trauma, to help individual family members to consider the needs of other family members, to build on people's strengths and to make positive changes to how the family operates as a whole.

Junior Doctors are medical doctors that are under the level of Consultant. The phrase 'junior doctors' includes doctors on the foundation level and more experienced speciality registrar levels. Within the Mental Health Team they work with supervision and support from Consultant Psychiatrists.

Both **Nurse Practitioners** and **Pharmacist Prescribers** provide vital access to quicker medication changes for patients with mental illnesses. These professionals will usually see patients that are moderately ill, rather than severely or critically mentally ill.

Occupational Therapists (OTs) are one of the most misunderstood, yet versatile and highly effective roles within the healthcare sector. As part of the Mental Health Team OTs help people to:

- Be independent by developing effective and practical coping strategies for day to day living. These activities may include cooking and eating, cleaning themselves and their home, doing their shopping, mobilising and getting to places and managing medications.
- Improve people's cognition and memory with a wide range of activities delivered over a number of sessions.

- Improve people's confidence and self-esteem.
- Identify other sources of support for people including support that could be offered by loved ones, professional services and voluntary services.

Pharmacists are experts in medicines. They know about pharmacokinetics, drug interactions, potential side effects, information about physical and mental illnesses and how herbal remedies can interact with medicines. They will often assist in medication reviews, helping Psychiatrists and patients with mental illnesses to get the best out of their medications with minimal or no side effects.

Physician Associates (or Physician Assistants) are new roles. They are there to support doctors. In Mental Health Teams they will assess people with mental illnesses, develop and review care plans. They are independent practitioners, but work under the supervision of doctors.

Play Therapists are often part of the multi-disciplinary team in Child & Adolescent Mental Health Services (CAMHS). Play is crucial for learning, expression of thoughts and feelings and in managing thoughts and feelings in children and young people. Play Therapists can be fundamental in supporting children and young people with mental illnesses.

Play Therapists will usually undertake an assessment based uniquely around play. Then deliver a number of therapy sessions.

Psychiatrists are Consultant level (the highest level) medical doctors that have significant experience of working with patients whom have mental illnesses. They work using the medical model. Psychiatrists often see and treat the most complex of patients with mental illnesses.

Psychologists (also known as Clinical Psychologists) deliver talking therapies aimed at changing the way people think, feel and behave. They are not medical doctors and work very differently.

People often get Psychiatrists and Psychologists mixed up or use the terms interchangeably due to lack of understanding about their different roles. Hopefully the descriptions above have clarified the distinct roles of the Psychiatrist and Psychologist.

Psychotherapists are Psychiatrists, Psychologists, CPNs or other Practitioners that have specialist training in psychotherapy. Psychotherapies includes the type of talking therapies discussed in Part 1 - Treatments & Recovery chapter of this book. But it might also other taking therapies such as Interpersonal Therapy, Dialectical Behaviour Therapy, Psychodynamic Therapy, Psychoanalysis, Supportive Therapy and Strengths-Based Therapy.

The role of **Social Workers** is diverse but is based on an holistic approach. It might involve giving safeguarding patients from harm or the risks of harm, advice around a wide range of topics, supporting patients to access services, assisting patients to apply for benefits, helping patients to engage with community social groups and ensure patients are supported to undertake their activities of daily living.

Support Workers (also known as Health Care Assistants or Clinical Support Workers) help other professionals in the multi-disciplinary team to care for patients with mental illnesses. This might include observation or monitoring of patients, follow up calls/appointments/home visits. Support Workers will usually work under the direct supervision of a Nurse, Doctor, Practitioner or other professional.

Team/Service Managers are responsible for ensuring the delivery of high quality, evidenced-based care that meets local, regional and national targets. They may have a service delivery background or not.

The 'S' Word

The 'S' Word - suicide - is the most taboo topic in mental illness. Everyone seems afraid to speak about it. I think it's partly because we are not sure what to say to someone experiencing suicidal thoughts and are worried about saying the wrong thing. But this lack of discussion only serves to further isolate those with suicidal ideation.

Let's start with some facts:

- Suicide is the biggest killer in men under the age of 45.
  (CALM, 2019)
- Suicide is the biggest killer in both men and women aged 20-34 years old.
  (Mental Health Foundation, 2019)
- Around 6,000 people take their own life every year in the UK.
  (Mental Health Foundation, 2019)
- A minimum of 20% of people will have suicidal thoughts over the course of their lifetime.
  (MIND, 2017)
- A minimum of 6.70% of people will attempt suicide over the course of their lifetime.
  (MIND, 2017)
- You are more at risk of suicidal thoughts if you have experienced adverse life events.
  (Patient, 2017)
- When someone gets suicidal thoughts, their brain is trying to reduce their stress levels and protect its self from damage.
  (Part 1 - Understanding, Mechanics of the Mind chapter of this book)

Thoughts of suicide might be fleeting and pass quite quickly, or be loud, repetitive and constant. For some people, suicidal thoughts become obsessional, meaning that they can't think about anything else.

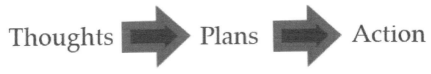

The Suicide Process

Thoughts ➡ Plans ➡ Action

There's no single reason that people decide to take their own lives or attempt to do so. But people who have survived a suicide attempt, report their reasons for the attempt as being:

- Unable to cope with destructive thought patterns.
- Unable to cope with negative emotions.
- Unable to tolerate the symptoms of mental illness any longer.
- Unable to deal with psychological pain caused by thoughts, feelings, memories or a combination of these causes.

People who have survived a suicide attempt still have to face the reasons for the attempt. Along with the additional thoughts and feelings that come as a result of their attempt.

They may feel shame or guilt having attempted to end their own lives. They may be fearful about the future and people they love finding out about the attempt. They may even be frustrated or angry that things didn't work out the way they had hoped.

Hopefully people that survive a suicide attempt get the treatment and support that they need. If someone discloses a suicide attempt to you, the best way to handle it is as follows:

- Reassure them that they won't be judged and don't judge them.
- Thank them for choosing to share this with you.
- Tell them that you recognise the courage it must have taken them to share this with you.
- Ask them what they would like to happen next.
- Ask them about current suicidal thoughts or plans.
- Ask them how they feel about the experience now.
- Always be honest. If they tell you something and you are unsure how to react, tell them this. Meaningful relationships are developed through honesty, trust and vulnerability.

Occasionally I have the odd suicidal thought. I disregard it, easily, as soon as I think it. But when I was really ill...it was a different story.

I remember spending hours thinking that suicide was the only way to end the torturous mood swings. I thought about a range of different ways to end my own life. I utilised my knowledge of how the body works to come up with the quickest and most pain-free way.

On the night of my life hiatus (see previous My Life Hiatus - Inpatient Admission chapter), I had a choice. I could either take a taxi to my local supermarket to pick up a sharp knife and then come home. Or I could tell the taxi driver to take me to my local A&E Department. I chose the latter.

Looking back on that choice now, without any doubt, it saved my life. It was also one of the best choices that I've ever made.

One More Thing About Suicide
Those that have lost someone they love due to suicide may have lots of questions.

Including: Why? Is there anything I could have done to prevent it? Why didn't I spot that something was wrong?

The best way to deal with these questions and the intense emotions associated with these questions is to seek the help of a professional counsellor.

References
CALM (2019) *'CALM - Suicide'* https://www.thecalmzone.net/help/get-help/suicide/, Last accessed on: 2nd February 2019.

Mental Health Foundation (2019) *'Mental Health Foundation - Suicide'* https://www.mentalhealth.org.uk/a-to-z/s/suicide, Last accessed on: 2nd February 2019.

MIND (2017) *'Mental Health Facts and Statistics'* https://www.mind.org.uk/information-support/types-of-mental-health-problems/statistics-and-facts-about-mental-health/how-common-are-mental-health-problems/, Last accessed on: 2nd February 2019.

Patient (2017) *'Dealing with Suicidal Thoughts'* https://patient.info/health/depression-leaflet/suicidal-

<u>thoughts</u>, last accessed: 2nd February 2019.

Poem: Sometimes High, Sometimes Low
Three years after my Life Hiatus, I've written something to reflect on the experience. Here it is, called *Sometimes High, Sometimes Low*:

Sometimes High, Sometimes Low

My thoughts race, I can do anything.

I am joyous, I feel like a king.

I get so much done.

Even cleaning out the kitchen cupboards is fun.

Am I losing my mind?

Guilt, despair and hopelessness feel intertwined.

I never want to leave my bed.

I am exhausted and have pain in my back, stomach and head.

Sometimes high, Sometimes low.

What will come next? I don't know.

I may do much, I may do nothing, just to get through the day.

I'm so tortured, desperate and powerless that I even pray.

I get a glimpse of being okay.

It gives me hope that come out of this I may.

I eat, bathe and move.

I ask for help, without it, I would never improve.

My life as I've known it is at an end.

It is time for me to reinvent myself and transcend.

I take medication, relax and check in with myself to keep well.

I never want to go through that again, it was like a living Hell.

Psychosis

Psychosis is an episode of losing touch with reality. People in an episode of psychosis don't always know that what they are experiencing isn't reality. Psychotic episodes might be positive, negative or mixed experiences. Signs & Symptoms of psychosis include:

- Visual, audio and tactile hallucinations - seeing things or people that others don't and aren't really there, hearing voices (these maybe hostile or friendly), feeling that things are touching you when nothing is, for example feeling that spiders are crawling all over your skin.
- Delusions - Having an idea or belief that isn't shared by others. For example, people in psychosis may believe that they are a super hero or God. People with delusions often come with thoughts or beliefs that someone is trying to harm or murder them.
- Speaking quickly and stumbling over words - caused by racing and fleeting thoughts.
- Paranoia.
- A wide range of emotional extremes: fear, panic, sadness, guilt, jealousy, despair, euphoria.
- Major disruption to day to day life, an inability to work during an episode and damage to interpersonal relationships.

I've never had a psychotic episode. The closest I've come in the height of my mental illness symptoms was to be convinced that I would win the Euro Millions Lottery. I would spend hours obsessing over what it will feel like when I have the winning ticket in my hand and check the numbers.

I felt how good it would be to never have to work again. I made detailed plans to spend whatever the estimated jackpot was. I accepted as fact that I would win. There was no doubt in my mind. No logical balanced thinking to explain the unrealistic odds.

I simply could not comprehend that my ticket wasn't a winning one. Just to give you the odds of winning the jackpot on the Euro Millions Lottery, it's over 36 million to 1, not that this fact mattered to my delusional mind. It would take me days of misunderstanding to finally realise and accept that I hadn't won. *This week*, my mind would tell me. I'd definitely win next week, I'd think over and over again. Then I'd go and buy more Euro Millions Lottery tickets and the pattern of thinking would start again.

Treatment for a psychotic episode usually starts with the person having the psychotic episode being admitted to a mental health ward. There they get given a range of medications and talking therapies to end the psychotic episode.

People who have experienced psychosis can usually remember the episode and tell you what they were thinking and how they felt. They can also recognise in retrospect what wasn't real, based on logical and balanced thinking. It's strange that psychosis usually seems to improve memory and memory recall.

Everyone is an individual and as such, some may not remember their episode of psychosis and rely on the memories of those around them.

Terrible Tolerance and Waiting

If you take medication for anything, including mental illness, over a long period of time your brain and body develops a tolerance. This means that the medication becomes less effective.

How long a tolerance takes to develop depends on the individual. You may get a tolerance quickly (weeks or months of use) or slowly (years or decades of use). The process of developing a tolerance is *so* gradual that you might not notice straight away. In fact, it might take you quite some time to understand that the symptoms of your illness are returning and that you need to have your medication reviewed. Here is a line graph that shows drug effectiveness over time:

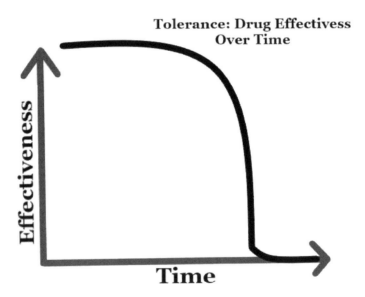

Tolerance: Drug Effectivess Over Time

When your brain and body develop a tolerance, you have two options:

1. Increase the dose of your medication.

2. Change your medication.

Any increases in dose or changes to your medication should be done under medical supervision. Some medications have withdrawal effects, which you may experience if you suddenly stop or decrease the dose too rapidly. The withdrawal symptoms range from relatively mild to extremely severe.

I am on a Quetiapine, a mood stabiliser medication. Developing a tolerance to this medication is beyond terrible. It's awful, frustrating and occasionally overwhelming. At times it feels like the mood swings are returning and that I am being tortured.

I visited my GP and explained how I was feeling in mood. My GP referred me to the Community Mental Health Team. I waited 4 weeks for a twenty-minute telephone assessment.

I was passed onto a Pharmacist Prescriber, another 4 week wait. She appeared to be concerned about hypomanic symptoms that I'm experiencing including:

- High levels of anxiety.
- Increased energy.
- Difficulties in falling or staying asleep.
- Increased productivity.
- Obsessional thinking.
- Being very irritable and frustrated.
- Switching between tasks without finishing any of them.

- Increase in desire to have sex.
- Feeling on edge and being unable to relax.
- Writing a lot.
- Fidgeting.
- Regular severe mixed mood states a couple of times per week.

Although many of these symptoms may seem positive at first glance, when your mind takes them to extremes, they become destructive and are damaging to your physical and mental health.

The Pharmacist Prescriber doubled the doses of my mood stabilising medication. This proved ineffective. She discussed my case with she with a Consultant Psychiatrist whom wants to see me. Another 5 week wait.

All this time waiting and struggling. All this time of lacking a quality of life. I can't even sleep off the symptoms.

I totally understand how underfunded the NHS is and in particular how under resourced mental health services are. So far I've waited 13 weeks (3 months and 1 week).

The wait feels eternal and I am beginning to feel that nothing will ever change. I know rationally that neither these last two emotionally driven thoughts are correct. Yet it can be difficult to disregard how you feel.

A Tale of Overcoming Adversity

I've wanted to write this for a long time. I've started it countless times, looking at adversity from many different angles. In the end, I decided that the best way to express what I want to say about adversity and overcoming adversity is through a little tale.

Growing up I had difficulties with reading and writing because of Dyslexia and Dyspraxia. At sixteen years old, I had a reading and comprehension age of fourteen. I remember when I was younger, having to read paragraphs two or three times to *get* the meaning of the words. The thought of reading a book at this age, was like the thought of climbing a mountain.

I couldn't write my name until I was ten years old. I understood what we were taught in classes, but just couldn't write it down on paper in an organised and structured way. I got very good at talking and verbal presentation to compensate.

Fast forward to now. I have overcome adversity in relation to reading and writing. I'm always reading at least ten books at any one time. I regularly get sent books by publisher's publicists to read and review on my blog.

Thankfully I no longer need to re-read paragraphs two or three times to understand them. I write creatively on a regular basis, have published short stories, have written for an online magazine and have written this book.

In addition to the above: I have done well academically. I have been to university three times. I have gained a Higher Education Diploma in Children's Nursing and an Honours

Degree in Nursing, graded at a 2:1, and successfully completed a Contraception: Theory & Practice module at Masters level.

The reading, the writing and the university wouldn't have been possible without overcoming adversity. But what's *really* interesting, is that I've learned some fundamental things that are required in order for anyone to overcome adversity. These include:

- Grit or determination. Not giving up.
- The support of others.
- Practice. Repetition is the key to learning and the way of getting good at anything. Think of when you learned to ride a bike as a child.
- Being driven by love or passion.
- People having belief and faith in you.
- Believing in yourself.

I wanted to share these thoughts, for anyone currently struggling with adversity. If you have overcome adversity, how did you do it? What did you need in order to overcome adversity?

Inspirational Quotes About Mental Health

Here are some inspirational quotes about mental health:

"What mental health needs is more sunlight, more candour, and more unashamed conversation."
- Glenn Close

"There is no health without mental health; mental health is too important to be left to the professionals alone, and mental health is everyone's business."
- Vikram Patel

"You are no less or more of a man or a woman or a human for having depression than you would be for having cancer or cardiovascular disease or a car accident,"
- Matt Haig

"If you are going through hell, keep going."
- Winston Churchill

"This feeling will pass. The fear is real but the danger is not."
- Cammie McGovern

"Sometimes the people around you won't understand your journey. They don't need to, it's not for them."
- Joubert Botha

"There is hope, even when your brain tells you there isn't."

- John Green

"It is during our darkest moments that we focus to see the light."
- Aristotle

"Knowing your own darkness is the best method for dealing with the darkness of other people."
- Carl Jung

"It's up to you today to start making healthy choices. Not choices that are just healthy for your body, but healthy for your mind"
- Steve Maraboli

"It doesn't have to take over your life, it doesn't have to define you as a person, it's just important to ask for help. It's not a sign of weakness."
- Demi Lovato

"You'll have bad times, but it'll wake you up to the good stuff you weren't paying attention to."
- Robin Williams

"Show up as the real you. The airbrushed you isn't sustainable, or even half as awesome."
- Kristen Lee Costa

"The world needs you even if you don't think it does. I promise, we need you here, now."

- Jason Manford

"You, yourself, as much as anybody in the entire universe, deserve your love and affection.'

- Buddha

Part 3 - Life Hacks

Self-Care

Self-care is anything that you do to look after your health. Self-care is about maintaining and preventing ill health. Health includes: physical, mental, emotional, social, environmental, financial and spiritual. Self-care should be part of your everyday life and it is essential for you to have good health.

Here are some examples of self-care:

Physical: nutritious meals, regular bathing, regular exercise, good amount and quality of sleep and medications for physical health problems.

Mental: talking therapies, meditation or mindfulness, coping strategies, distraction activities, relaxation and medications for mental illnesses.

Emotional: processing and dealing with feelings, expressing of feelings, allowing time for emotional healing. Letting go of worry, recognising and managing fear.

Social: catching up with family and friends, professional relationships at work, recognising when you need time to yourself and taking it.

Environmental: cleaning, decluttering, spending time in nature and places of beauty.

Financial: being aware of income and expenditure, paying bills, saving up for big items or experiences, paying off debt.

Spiritual: spending time in places spiritually significant form you - this might be churches or in nature, spending time with religious or spiritual leaders, other practises you associate with your spiritual well-being.

There's nothing selfish self-care. It's about keeping yourself healthy. Self-care isn't always easy either. Sometimes in order to care for yourself you have to say no to other people's wants and needs.

Other times you might be faced with difficult decisions about your lifestyle, working patterns or income in order to make more time for self-care activities.

Reflect on your daily routine. How many activities are related to self-care? Do you need to build more self-care into your daily, weekly or monthly routines? Only you will know the answers to these questions.

This part of the book, Life Hacks, is all about self-care.

The Well of Resilience

Resilience or *emotional resilience* is our ability to deal with adverse events in life that cause pressure or stress. I like to think of resilience as being like water in a well:

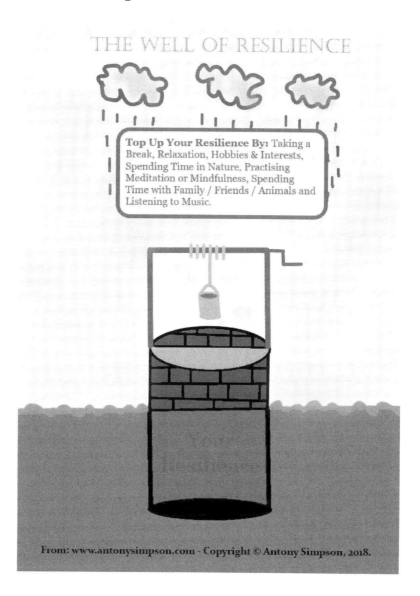

THE WELL OF RESILIENCE

Top Up Your Resilience By: Taking a Break, Relaxation, Hobbies & Interests, Spending Time in Nature, Practising Meditation or Mindfulness, Spending Time with Family / Friends / Animals and Listening to Music.

From: www.antonysimpson.com - Copyright © Antony Simpson, 2018.

We only have so much resilience within us, like there is only so much water in a well. Adverse events cause us to use our resilience water by the bucket loads. But there is good news.

We can make it rain to add more resilience water to the well at any time. We can do this by: Taking a Break, Relaxation, Hobbies & Interests, Spending Time in Nature, Practising Meditation or Mindfulness, Spending Time with Family / Friends / Animals and Listening to Music.

10 Easy Ways to Improve Your Mental Health
Here's 10 easy ways to improve your mental health:

10. Regular Exercise
I don't mean becoming a gym bunny or taking up running. Start walking. Walking is the easiest form of exercise. Take it slow and easy. Do it regularly, a couple of times a week. Gradually build up the distance. It's even better if you can walk in places of natural beauty, as you'll have the scenery to enjoy as well.

NHS Choices says:

"Research shows that physical activity can also boost self-esteem, mood, sleep quality and energy, as well as reducing your risk of stress, depression..."

(From: NHS Choices, last accessed: Thursday 28th September 2017)

9. A Better Diet
We could all do with eating a bit better right? Add more fruit and vegetables to your diet – aim for five a day. Cut down on the amount of sugar and salt in your food. Try to drink 6-8 glasses of fluid per day (roughly 1.2 litres). You can learn more about diet on the NHS Choices – Eatwell Guide website.

8. Go Smoke-Free
Despite many smokers saying that a cigarette reduces their stress levels, Nicotine is a stimulant drug which means it has the opposite effect. It increases anxiety and stress levels, especially when those nicotine receptors in the brain need feeding. Becoming smoke-free has loads of other benefits as well.

7. Drink Less Alcohol
Alcohol is a depressant drug and affects your brain chemistry.

Drinking a small amount of alcohol decreases inhibitions and can make you feel happier. But <u>drinking heavily can lead to a lowered mood</u>. It's also not a good idea to drink if you are angry or upset, as it can make you feel worse and you might do things that you wouldn't do sober.

You don't have to stop drinking alcohol, just cut down on the amount. A good tip is to buy less alcohol. If you buy less alcohol you'll have less to drink.

6. Meditation or Mindfulness

<u>Research</u> suggests that daily meditation for just 20 minutes per day has benefits to mental health after just five days. Benefits of meditation include: lower stress levels, feeling more positive, improved concentration, improves the ability to be in the moment and helps with clarity of thought. You can learn more about the practice of meditation and mindfulness in Part 1 - Treatments & Recovery chapter of this book.

5. Recognise the Signs of Stress

Recognise when your stressed and take steps to relax. You can do this by taking a deep breath, focusing on your body, thoughts and feelings and look for signs of stress. I call this checking-in with myself and try to do it at least a few times a day. The signs of stress can be found in Part 1 - A List of Common Conditions chapter of this book.

4. It's okay to say NO

When we think about saying no to people, we imagine the world will end. But the reality is nothing like our imagination. In fact, most of the time, people are okay about it. Remember that it is okay to say no and say it when you need to do so. Sometimes it's better to say no rather than say yes. Otherwise we risk over committing ourselves and spread our limited energy too thinly.

3. Sleep

Sleep is *so* important for good mental health. Sleep allows our bodies to rest and repair. The average adult needs eight hours of sleep. But children and teenagers need much more. But it's not just about the amount of the sleep you get, it's also about the quality. Poor quality sleep lowers resilience and increases the risk of physical and mental illness. Get your shut-eye in and try to have a good sleep routine.

2. Off-Load

We all need people to talk to and to off-load to at times. Some off-load to their families, their spouses, their friends or their therapists. Find some people in your life who you can off-load to.

Important characteristics in people you choose to off-load to: they should give you a feeling of trust, they should have the ability to actively listen to what you say, they should be non-judgemental, they should be empathetic and they should challenge you when needed.

1. Relaxation

Write a list of things that help you relax. Then do some of the things on the list on a regular basis. For example, reading really relaxes me. So every night before bed, I read, even if it's just for ten minutes.

References

NHS Choices – Benefits of exercise
NHS Choices – Eatwell Guide
Smokefree NHS
Drink Aware – Alcohol and mental health

NHS Choices – Does meditation reduce stress?
NHS Choices – How to deal with stress
One You – Sleep

Tips to Help You Deal with Worry and Anxiety

Recognising that you're anxious is the first step to addressing it.

Overwhelmed ANGST www.antonysimpson.com

Anxiety NERVOUS Alarmed

Apprehension Worry Fustration

Pain in the neck uncertainty

Tense Out of My Control PANIC!

Here are the signs and symptoms of anxiety:

Effects of anxiety in your body:

- Feeling like a tightly coiled spring.
- Aches and pains - including headaches, back pain and stomach pain.
- Being fidgety - unable to sit still.
- A feeling of heaviness in the pit of your stomach.
- Uncontrollable sweating, when the room is at a cool temperature.
- Breathing faster, shallow breathing or forgetting to take a deep breath.
- Difficulty in sleeping - either getting to sleep or staying to sleep (insomnia).
- A fast heart beat - it beating so fast that you can feel it in your head or near your ears.
- Feeling nauseous.
- Needing to go to the toilet more or less often.
- Having panic attacks.

Effects of anxiety in your mind:

- Worrying or feeling like your worrying is out of control. You could be worrying about anything including: work, children, relationships, money, the future.
- Rumination or a constant critical inner voice (see Part 2 - Rumination & Critical Inner Voice chapter of this book for more information).
- Finding it difficult to relax or being unable to do so.
- Feeling overwhelmed.
- Paranoia - Thinking that others can spot your anxiety, or that they think negatively of you.
- A sense of dread and always expecting the worst.
- Derealisation - Feeling a sense of disconnection from the world and people around you. It's like feeling that nothing is real.
- Seeking excessive reassurance that you haven't upset the people around you.
- Seeking excessive reassurance that your behaviours or actions are acceptable to others.

There's lots of advice out there about what you can do to deal with worry and anxiety. But what actually helped me deal with my worry and anxiety? Doing these:

1. Off-load to a supportive friend – This gave a voice to my worries. The simple act of telling someone helped me sort through my worries and realise what was and wasn't within my control.
2. Remind yourself what is outside of your control – I was worried about a lot of things outside of my

control. It helped to remind myself to try not to worry about things I had no control over. That I should focus on addressing things that were within my control.

3. Double or triple relaxation time – This was something I did to reduce my heightened stress levels because of the worry and anxiety. At first, I did feel guilty spending so much of my time relaxing. But each time I felt guilty, I reminded myself that this self-care was essential in order to prevent mental illness.

4. Distraction – This is something I did repeatedly during my relaxation time. Intruding thoughts and emotions of worry and anxiety would often enter my head and it was my job to ignore those thoughts and distract myself from them.

5. Write down all worries – It helped to get the worries out of my head where they were going around and around like a CD stuck on repeat. It also put my worries into perspective, helped me face them and sort through them. This cleared my mind, giving me clarity that allowed me to start planning what needed to be done. Anyone that's been worried or anxious will know that the emotions make it difficult to think clearly. So this strategy was really helpful.

22 Relaxing Activity Ideas

Being able to relax is a skill, one that can be learned with practice. It's like learning to ride a bike. You will need to practice relaxing often to get good at it. A relaxation routine can help, as our brain's like patterns of behaviour.

Here are some ideas of activities that can help you to relax. Try using a couple of them in combination to create a relaxation routine:

22. TV, Films or Netflix.
Watch something you can enjoy but that isn't too emotionally provoking or too taxing on the mind.

21. Watch some comedy.
Something that makes you laugh-out-loud. Laughing can be a great way to reduce tension and help you to relax.

20. Go for a walk in a place of natural beauty.
Walking in nature is scientifically proven to increase levels of serotonin and dopamine and reduce levels of cortisol. If you can't get out to a place of natural beauty look at photos or images of a place of natural beauty. Consider setting a photo of natural beauty as a wallpaper or lock screen on your phone.

19. Take a day off social media and use your phone sparingly.
Try to live without it for a whole 24 hours, if that's possible. The constant notifications on phones can make us feel stressed or anxious.

18. Massage.

A professional masseur can work wonders! But it doesn't have to be a professional. If you have a romantic partner, they can give you a massage. Just remember to give them lots of positive verbal feedback about what you like. Experiment. You and your partner could start with a scalp massage, or with shoulders and back before proceeding on to full body massages. A tip here: use baby oil to enhance the experience, just remember to put down towels beforehand.

17. Listen to music.

Listen to any type of music that has a slow and relaxing beat, rhythm and vocals. You could even put a relaxation playlist together.

16. Fresh bedding and pyjamas.

Sometimes, with life being so busy, we forget about the little things that really help us to unwind and relax. Put fresh bedding on, have a long bath or shower and then put on clean pyjamas. You'll feel like you're in relaxation heaven when you get into bed.

15. Burn scented candles or essential oils.

Relaxing essential oil scents include: jasmine, sandalwood, ylang-ylang, patchouli, rose, lavender, chamomile, lilac and vanilla. Just remember to never leave a lit candle unattended. It wouldn't be very relaxing to have your house catch fire!

14. Reading.

Reading can aid relaxation. Especially if it's as part of a relaxation routine. Try to get in the habit of reading for 15-30 minutes a day before bed. Over time you'll gradually realise that as soon as you pick up a book your whole body starts to relax and unwind. I try to do this every evening before bed.

13. Take a nap.
Listen to your body. If your body is telling you that it's tired or worse exhausted, take a short nap. The benefits of napping on physical and mental health have been evidenced through research. Like everything moderation is key. Don't have a long nap, as it will make you feel more tired and may disrupt your body clock and normal sleeping pattern.

12. Double the time you think it will take to do a task.
We often under estimate the time it will take us to do a task. Then we get stressed trying to get it done in the tight timescale. Doubling the time you think it will take you to do a task, is not only giving yourself a more realistic timescale, it might leave you with some spare time. If you happen to have some spare time after you complete your task, use it to reward yourself by doing something enjoyable.

This will leave you less pressured as it's probably a more realistic timescale.

11. Mediate or practice mindfulness.
Both mediation and mindfulness have been discussed in detail in Part 1 - Treatments & Recovery chapter of this book. They're evidenced through countless scientific studies to improve short term relaxation, long term ability to relax quickly and with ease and to reduce levels of stress.

10. Book a holiday.
Taking a break from the stress of everyday life is really important. It doesn't have to be expensive and it doesn't have to be abroad. The key concept here is to *escape*. If you

take a week off work, but stay at home, you will end up doing things that you would normally fit into your everyday life. Yes, it's good to get on top of things, but you will find you don't take that break. Whereas if you are away from home you have escaped day to day life, you can properly loosen up and slow down.

9. Clear the clutter.

Tidy up. Clear away the clutter. Put everything back in its place. You'll feel better not having to navigate or working around the clutter.

8. Go for a Reiki treatment.

Reiki is a form of energy that is in everything in the universe, including in our aura or soul. In a reiki treatment, a Reiki Practitioner tops up your energy with reiki energy from the universe. They channel the energy into you and the reiki energy goes to where it is needed. Reiki is used as a complementary therapy to help people with all sorts of chronic illnesses and diseases to relax. People include cancer patients and patients receiving end of life care.

7. Sunbathe.

Sunbathing is subject to weather. In the UK we probably don't get enough sunlight. Sunlight is a great source of Vitamin D. Vitamin D improves mood, helps with weight loss and helps to strengthen bones. If you live in a climate like the UK, you can take Vitamin D supplements. If you are on any medications, you should discuss taking Vitamin D supplements with your GP before doing so.

6. Spend time with pets.

Spending time with pets can really be beneficial for both the owner and the pet.

I have two gorgeous Bengal cats, Russell and Dylan:

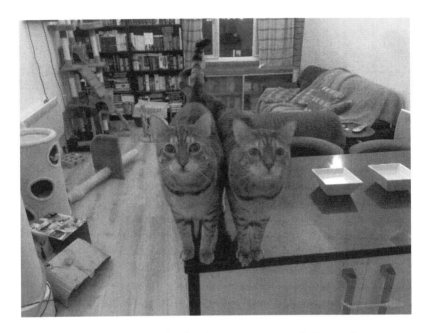

Bengal cats are known for being more vocal than the average house cats. I just didn't realise quite *how* vocal they could be. They have this awful high-pitched meowing that they do whenever they want something including: food, water and attention. This meowing puts me on edge. It isn't a relaxing sound in the slightest. So I deliberately don't give my cats attention when they are meowing, only when they are quiet, giving positive reinforcement for the behaviour I want.

The moral of the story? If a pet makes you on edge with its behaviour or has behaviour that is difficult to manage, it's probably learned behaviour. The good news is that with time and training you can change your pet's behaviour. That written, never expect an animal to behave in a different way than its instincts dictate.

Bengal cats have always been more vocal than average house cats, this is a fact I'm never going to be able to change. Nor is the fact that the high-pitched meow mimics the cry of a new born baby and has been honed by cats over centuries to get food, water and attention from humans. All I can do is minimise the behaviour by rewarding them with attention when they are quiet.

5. Adult colouring books.

Adult colouring books are a great distraction from the trials and tribulations of everyday life. Plus they're fun!

4. Catch up with friends and off-load.

Spend time with people who are positive, emotionally warm and who you can connect with on an intimate level. There are loads of benefits to off-loading that have been written about in previous chapters.

3. Go out to your favourite restaurant for tea.

Your favourite meal. A good atmosphere. Good company. What better way to take it easy?

2. Take an extra-long piping hot bath.

Include some luxury bubble bath, body wash and shampoo.

1. A nice cup of Tea.

Probably because I'm British, but a nice cup of tea instantly relieves stress and helps me to breathe and to take a moment to relax.

9 Reasons to Keep A Gratitude Journal

A gratitude journal is a diary were you write a list of the things you are grateful for each day. There are many good reasons to keep a Gratitude Journal. Here are 9 reasons:

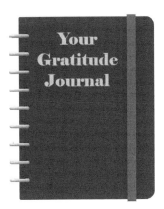

1. Changes Your Mindset

We're hardwired to be alert for threats and danger. This means that our default mindset is negative. Keeping a gratitude journal changes your mindset to a positive one, by focusing on the things you are grateful for.

2. Find More Happiness Everyday

The practice of gratitude journaling helps you spot little moments of happiness throughout the day that you might otherwise miss.

3. Challenges Negative Self-Beliefs

Keeping any sort of journal increases your self-awareness. You might discover you hold some negative self-beliefs. You can use the journal to challenge negative self-beliefs.

4. Good for Reflecting

A gratitude journal helps you reflect on a wide range of topics including: what makes you happy, what stresses you out, how you think, feel and behave, how others treat you, the bigger picture, the learning of the day, and what you could do differently in the future,

5. Reflecting Can Be Relaxing

Offloading all of your thoughts, feelings and behaviours into a journal can take the pressure out of your head and onto the page (or screen). It can help you to let go and relax.

6. Increases Your Confidence

A gratitude journal increases your confidence by helping you to recognise what you do well and your successes in life.

7. A Tool to Improve Relationships

A gratitude journal can improve relationships by focusing on the good things people do for you and the good things you do for others. It isn't about the big things (like buying someone a car or engagement ring), it's about the many little things that combine to make a big difference.

Little things can include: considering you, helping you out with household tasks, messaging to see how you are, allowing you to offload, sharing dreams, desires and fears, getting clothes out for you, running you a bath, giving you a kiss and a cuddle, appreciating your talents and skills, giving you compliments, letting you choose what both of you watch on the TV, the list is endless.

8. A Tool to Set and Keep Track of Goals

A journal allows you to write down a list of goals and track the progress you make towards these goals on a daily basis.

9. Entries can be as Short or Long as You Want

There are no rules to keeping a gratitude journal. You can make entries as short or as long as you want. It need not be a big task. Just 5 minutes at the end of the day.

There are no downsides to keeping a gratitude journal. It is well worth doing.

Tips for a Better Night's Sleep

Sleep is essential for our body and mind. The functions of sleep and resulting benefits include:

- Helps the body to restore and repair. Blood pressure drops, muscles become relaxed, tissue growth and repair occurs, improves the immune response and immune system.
- Helps the brain to process information and store memory.
- Helps the brain function normally when awake.
- Increases concentration, decision making abilities and social skills when awake.
- Enhances creativity when awake.
- Reduces stress by lowing levels of cortisol.
- Reduces likelihood of gaining weight.
- Reduces likelihood of impulsive thoughts or behaviours when awake.
- Reduces likelihood of requiring stimulants to keep you awake during the day (e.g. caffeine, nicotine).
- Reduces likelihood of requiring sedatives to help you get to and stay a sleep (e.g. alcohol and sleeping tablets).
- Makes waking up, ready to start the day much easier.

Children and young people need around 9-11 hours of sleep. The average adult needs 8 hours of sleep. Elderly people need 8 hours of sleep, but split up into naps. These are all averages. Every person is unique, some people need more or less sleep than others. To find out how much sleep you need, check in with your body and listen to it.

The best way to get a good night's sleep is to have a sleep routine. A pattern of behaviours or rituals that are completed every night before you go to bed. These behaviours or rituals become associated with going to sleep.

For example, my sleep routine includes: reducing the light in my bedroom a short time before I go to bed, reading for at least half an hour before putting my head on my pillow and then using meditation to clear my mind for 5 minutes (if I stay awake for long enough!) once in bed with the lights off.

Many people have times in their lives when they have difficulty with sleep. They may struggle to get to sleep or to stay asleep (insomnia) or may not get the quality sleep they require.

Here's some tips for a better night's sleep:

- Have a sleep routine. Try going to bed at the same time every night and waking up at the same time every morning.
- Make sure the bedroom is dimly lit before bed and dark during the night.
- Make the bedroom as quiet as possible at night.
- Make sure your mattress is comfortable, so comfortable that you look forward to going to bed.
- Don't have anything that will distract your mind or keep it awake in the bedroom.
- Ensure the bedroom is at a cool temperature - this is good for inducing sleep.
- Reduce light exposure for half an hour before bed. This includes limiting use of screens: laptops, TVs, iPads, etc.

- Relax before bed (see previous chapter titled 22 Great Ways to Relax for ideas).
- Try not to drink caffeine after midday (I know this is easier said than done, especially if you've had a run of nights with bad sleep).
- Avoid caffeine, nicotine, alcohol and drugs. They are all substances that are known to interfere with decent quality sleep.
- Seek out morning light.
- Don't get anxious when you can't sleep. This only makes your brain produce Noradrenaline and Cortisol, both of which are designed to keep you awake and alert.
- In fact, if you can't get to sleep after 30 minutes of trying, get up and do something else. Go back to bed when you feel sleepy.
- Use a Sleep Tracker App. These are useful at finding out what is going on when you're unconscious.
- If a pet is waking you up, ensure that they don't have access to the bedroom.
- See your GP if you are struggling to get a good night's sleep over a significant period of time. Your GP may refer you to a sleep clinic where your sleep problems will be investigated. You may have a condition like sleep apnoea. I know several people diagnosed with sleep apnoea. The treatment has transformed their sleep and enhanced the quality of their waking life.

Sleep well.

How to Deal with Difficult Emotions

There are lots of emotions that make us feel good, happy and content. These emotions make life an enjoyable experience and we often don't struggle with these emotions. They make the world a wonderful place to be in. But in this chapter, we will focus on dealing with the more difficult emotions.

Triggers

Emotions can be triggered by: stimuli (a situation, event or experience) or a chemical imbalance in the brain. They vary in intensity and duration. Sometimes they are transient passing quickly, and other times they stick with us for days, weeks, months or even years.

Here are some negative emotions and different levels of intensity:

Difficult Emotions

Frustration	Anger	Rage
Alarm	Fear	Panic
Apprehension	Anxiety	Dread/Terror
Upset	Wounded	Rejection
Boredom	Desperation	Contempt
Sadness	Sorrow/Despair	Grief
Dislike	Disgust	Revulsion
Confusion	Embarrassment	Humiliation
Regret	Guilt	Shame

Desire	Envy	Jealousy
Inadequate	Despondent	Depression
Solitary	Isolated	Lonely
Disorientation	Agitation	Confusion
Discontentment	Disappointment	Failure/Disaster
Alienation	Hatred	Cruelty
Helpless	Victimised	Persecuted
Hurt	Pain	Suffering
Tired	Fatigue	Exhausted

→

Level of Intensity

Identify How You Feel

To start with you need to identify how you are feeling and know why you are feeling this way. For example, *I am feeling frustrated. This is because...*

Some people choose to avoid difficult emotions. This isn't a good way to deal with difficult emotions. It can lead to unhealthy coping strategies, self-destructive and self-sabotage behaviours (such as over eating, smoking, drinking too much alcohol, using drugs and getting into debt due to over spending).

Accept How You Feel

Next you need to accept how you feel right now. If it's particularly difficult, remember that how you feel *will* change, our emotions are not permanent.

The best way to deal with a difficult emotion is to express the emotion in an appropriate way. There are lots of ways to do this, talking with family or friends, writing down how you feel, creating something. It's also better to express your emotion when at its lowest level of intensity. Otherwise the emotion may increase in intensity and get more difficult to deal with.

Some people choose not to express their emotions, particularly difficult ones. This bottling up of emotions is like an internal pressure cooker. If you don't let off steam from the internal pressure cooker by expressing your emotions, you'll eventually explode with an extremely intense negative emotion. This can be unpleasant for you and people around you.

Deal with the Emotion and Let It Go

The final step is to deal with the emotion before letting it go. Dealing with the emotion will depend on what emotion it is. But ways to deal with emotions include: increasing your Well of Resilience (see previous chapter The Well of Resilience), reframing your thinking (focus on the positives, practicing gratitude, increasing your kindness to yourself and others), distraction activities, relaxation techniques and talking therapies.

Sometimes difficult emotions or the situation, event or experience that triggered these emotions requires time to heal. The amount of time varies on the individual and the circumstances. Be kind and take good care of yourself while you heal.

Strengths-Based Decision-Making Model

Strengths-based talking therapy is focused on recognising the individual's strengths and resilience strategies in dealing with challenges. I've adapted strengths-based therapy to develop a Strengths-Based Decision-Making Model. The benefits of this model are:

- It focuses on the strengths of the individual. We are usually quick to identify our areas of development, but not to identify and recognise our strengths.
- Resilience strategies help us be prepared for when things don't go to plan.
- We identify the challenge and then all possible options. Our thinking can be in binary terms, meaning we only see a couple of solutions. This model encourages you to think of all the different options – including ones you wouldn't have normally considered.
- It encourages you to come up with a Plan of Action.
- If you use this model often enough, it will eventually become an automatic way of looking at challenges.

Here is an example of the model in practice:

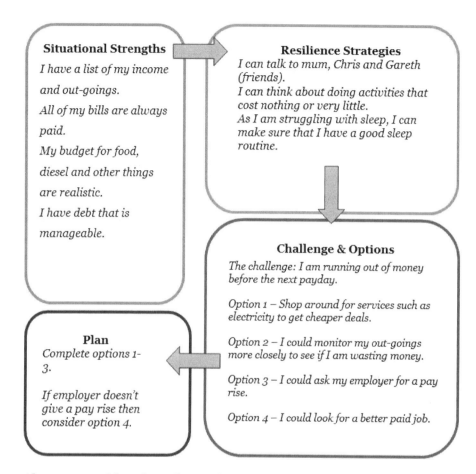

Always consider the what, why, how, who and by when:

- What can I do?
- Why is this challenge important?
- How can I deal with this challenge?
- How can I make best use of my strengths and resilience strategies?
- Who can support or help me?
- How can others support me?
- By when do actions on the plan needed to be completed?

On the next page you'll find the Strength-Based Decision-

Making Model to complete for yourself.

Strengths-Based Decision-Making Model

Use this model to identify your strengths and resilience strategies in thinking about how to deal with a challenge. Consider all possible options, then come up with a plan of action.

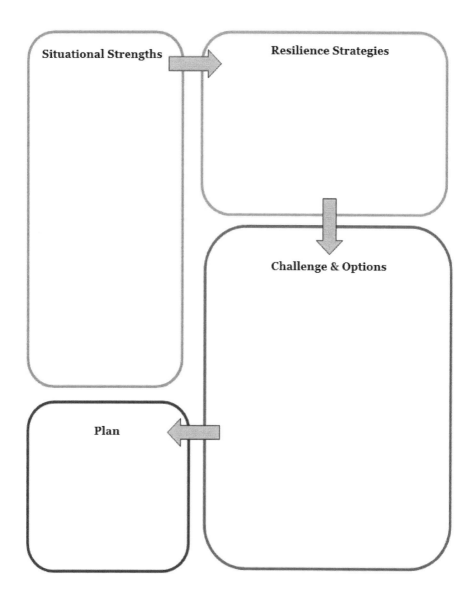

You can download a printer friendly version of this Strength-Based Decision-Making Model from:
www.mentalhealthwisdombook.com.
Copyright © Antony Simpson, 2019.

A List of Distraction Activities

Distraction Activities can prevent rumination, alleviate symptoms of mental illness and prevent boredom. Here are some ideas for distraction activities:

Acting. Arrange a family day out. Art therapy. Book a holiday. Buy yourself some flowers or a house plant. Change the music on your phone. Clean the house. Colour in your adult colouring book. Cook something. Create playlists around a variety of topics (including: friendship, love, mental health, songs associated with good memories, upbeat songs, motivation). Create your bucket list. Dance. Declutter. Do a crossword or puzzle. Do a jigsaw. Do a paint/colour in by numbers. Do some gardening. Do something nice for someone else. Do your clothes washing and drying. Drawing.

Find a bargain on eBay. Follow your curiosity – learn about something new. Get rid of any Apps you don't use on your phone or tablet. Go bowling. Go camping. Go clothes shopping. Go do yoga. Go food shopping. Go for a drive. Go for a hot air balloon ride. Go for a massage. Go for a picnic. Go for a pub lunch with a friend. Go for a reiki treatment. Go for a run. Go for a spar day. Go for a walk. Go away for the weekend. Go for coffee and cake with a friend. Go horse riding. Go on a city break. Go on a train journey. Go rock climbing. Go skiing. Go skydiving. Go to a concert. Go to a funfair or theme park. Go to a zoo. Go to bingo. Go to the cinemas. Go to the gym. Go to the park. Graphic design.

Have a chocolate treat. Have a Disney marathon. Have a film marathon. Have a nap. Have a snack. Have an extra-long bath. Join a drama group. Knitting. Learn a new language. Learn to play a musical instrument. Learn to play chess or checkers. Light a scented candle, or essential oil burner, enjoy the fragrance. Listen to Podcasts. Listen to music.

Look at the clouds, see what shapes and things you can see. Look through some old photos.

Make a cup of tea. Make a mocktail. Make a vision board. Meditate. Organise something (this could be your collection of books, music and films, both physical objects and electronic). Painting. Photography. Play a board game. Play a card game with someone. Play a computer game. Play a musical instrument. Play the 'would you rather … or …' game with a friend. Put together a Well-Being kit. Read up on psychology. Read up on the life of a celebrity. Reading. Rearrange furniture at home.

Sculpture. See a show at a theatre. Shop online. Sort through your Bits 'n' Pieces draw. Sort through the photos on your phone. Sort through your clothes. Spend time in a forest. Spend time with pets. Stargaze. Start a blog. Stay in and order a takeaway. Take a community college/evening course. Telephone or Face Time a friend. Text someone to tell them that you love them. Try some food you've never tried before.

Visit a beach. Visit a museum. Visit an animal sanctuary. Visit Ikea. Visit somewhere new. Volunteer. Watch Comedy. Watch Films. Watch something new on Netflix. Watch the most popular programme on the BBC iPlayer. Watch videos on YouTube. Water indoor plants. Write a poem. Write a short story. Write down 10 things you are good at. Write fan fiction. Write in your gratitude journal. Write product reviews on Amazon.

The Double Spirals of Selflessness and Selfishness
We all have two spirals within us. The selflessness spiral and the selfishness spiral:

The Double Spirals

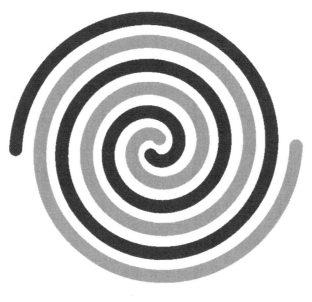

◻ Selflessness Spiral

◼ Selfishness Spiral

The selflessness spiral is all about considering the needs and wants of others. The behaviour includes activities that help and support others.

The selfishness spiral is all about considering your needs and wants. The behaviour includes activities that meet your needs and wants.

Neither spiral is good or bad. We need both spirals. The selflessness spiral is essential to caring for babies, children and others. The selfishness spiral is essential for self-care and remaining physically and mentally healthy.

These spirals need to be in balance. Being too selfless can lead to being taken advantage of and becoming a doormat. Being too selfish can lead to breakdown of relationships and becoming socially isolated.

It is difficult to get these two spirals in balance and to keep them there in life. Every day these spirals are challenged and often one takes precedence over the other. The benefits of having these two spirals in balance include:

- More balanced and fairer thinking.
- Preventing physical and mental illness by not working to the point of burnout.
- Preventing being taken advantage of.
- Preventing social isolation.
- Being more considerate of other people's needs.
- Increased empathy.
- Knowing when to take a step back and look after yourself.
- Increased self-awareness.
- Forward thinking - the ability to consider the consequences of a choice in the future.
- Increased assertiveness.

Think about the spirals within you. Do you tend to be more selfless or selfish? What can you change to promote balance?

Daily Mood Diary

Day:_____**Date:**_____

It is recommended that you complete a daily mood diary for at least two weeks in order to identify any patterns. Share this mood diary with your GP or Mental Health Team.

Time	Mood Rating (1 to 10)	Activity	Triggers
6:00-8:00			
9:00-11:00			
12:00-15:00			
16:00-18:00			
19:00-21:00			
22:00-23:00			
00:00-02:00			
03:00-05:00			

Mood Rating

Rate your mood using the following scale:

- **1** – The worst you've ever felt. Suicidal thoughts that are difficult to ignore. Feelings of depression: hopelessness, guilt, sadness or nothing. Impossible to do anything.
- **2-3** – Feeling low. Slow thinking or limited concentration span. Sleeping more or less than normal. Feelings of depression: hopelessness, guilt, sadness or nothing. Struggling to do daily tasks. May require breaks for hours at a time due to exhaustion following completion of a task.
- **4** – Feeling low. But you may be able to function in day to day life.
- **5** – Feeling neither good nor bad. Being able to do the activities of daily living.
- **6-8** – Feeling good. Really good. Optimistic, very productive. Doing everything to excess: talking, tasks and are super social. May flip from task to task without completing them.
- **9** – Feeling amazing. High levels of confidence in yourself. Rapid thinking and talking. Feeling good for no reason or despite things going on in your life. Very creativity and full of ideas.
- **10** – The best you've ever felt. You feel like you can do anything. You may begin to hallucinate or think/feel things that are not real. You may spend ridiculous amounts of money.

You can download a printer friendly version of this mood diary from: <u>www.mentalhealthwisdombook.com</u>.

Copyright © Antony Simpson, 2019.

How to support someone with Mental Illness

Supporting someone with mental illness can be difficult. What should you say and not say? What should you do and not do?

First educate yourself around mental illness. Mental health charities Mind and SANE both have informative websites.

Second: **You must look after yourself**. You can't support anyone else if you are not physically, mentally or emotionally well.

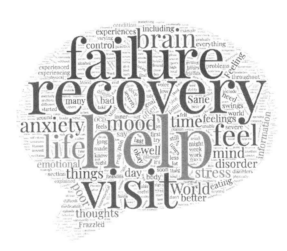

The practical advice to support someone with mental illness:

- Stay in contact with them. Ask them *how* they would like you to keep in contact. Some may prefer phoning or seeing; whereas others may prefer messaging or texting.

- Unconditional love and care. Let them know that you love them unconditionally and care for them deeply. Don't have any expectation that they will reciprocate.
- Listen to what they say and don't assume anything.
- Ensure that there are no distractions when you are with them or on the phone to them. Put your phone on silent and make sure any loud children are pets are out of the way (if you have them).
- Offer practical support. Go shopping for them or with them, help them to clean, cook them a meal. Whatever it is that they need. They may be resistant to the idea of practical help, so reassure them that you are happy to help and that you know they'd do it for you.
- Remind them to take their medication or when appointments are due. People with mental illness tend to have poor short-term memories.
- Ask them about their appetite and diet. If they have an appetite but are struggling to make anything (due to lack of energy and/or motivation), find out what their favourite meal is and cook it for them.
- Offer distracting activities. Distracting activities that you can both do together can give someone a break from their own critical inner of voice. The activities can be something as simple as a walk around the park. Make sure you are always led by the person with mental illness though. If they say that they are too unwell or tired to do the activity, don't take it personally. And certainly don't judge them or take offence.
- Help them access support. This could include going with them to their GP, counselling sessions or mental

health service appointments. Offer to sit in appointments with them, but let them know that it's okay if they want to be seen alone.

- Be understanding. Someone with mental illness may cancel plans at the last minute. You may arrive at their house to find it messy and them disheveled. Don't take it personally, let them know that you understand and ask if there is any way that you can help.

- Be patient. Like any illness, mental illness takes the right treatment, the right support and *time* for them to start to feel better.

- Limit questions and time spent with them, if you feel they are exhausted and need to rest. You'll be able to spot if they need to rest by: pulling on their hair, forgetting what you've just said to them, being very slow to respond, unable to think of words, dropping of their head, shuffling of feet and other body language people use when they look like they are about to drop off to sleep.

- Be aware of your own body language and theirs. Try and display open body language and avoid mirroring.

- Try not to give advice, as often it is unrealistic and unhelpful. For example, never advise someone with depression to exercise more or have a healthier diet. This person has probably used all of their energy and motivation to get out of the bed. This single action has left them more exhausted than they have ever been in their life. So advising them to exercise, eat an healthier diet or make big changes to their life will seem unachievable and may come across as if you are blaming them for their mental illness.

- Sign-post them to useful resources. Such as: <u>NHS Choices</u>, <u>Time to Change</u>, <u>Mental Health Foundation</u>, <u>Mind</u>, <u>SANE</u>, <u>Anxiety UK</u> and <u>Bipolar UK</u>.

How to Be Kinder

Kindness is being friendly or generous to others. It's showing understanding, empathy and sympathy towards others. Considering and completing acts that help or assist another, without the expectation of anything in return.

The world needs more kindness, so here are some ways to be kinder:

- Be kind, friendly and compassionate to everyone you interact with. Whether you perceive them as being in need of kindness or not. Even if they are the complete opposite with you.
- Pay people genuine and authentic compliments.
- Drop the judgement - of other people and yourself.
- Learn about kindness from others. Go through your memory and remember times people were kind to you. How did they behave? Try imitating some of this behaviour.
- View your kindness as a strength. Make kindness a value that you live your life by.
- Meditate with your focus on kindness.
- Point out kindness in others, encourage them to keep being kind and congratulate them for it.
- Be present and in the moment. See more, hear more, touch more, taste more and smell more. The more you sense the more you are likely to see kindness in others.
- Don't expect perfection from yourself or others. Recognise that we are all doing our best and that we are all human.

- Use your manners. Say please and thank you. You would be surprised how kind and respectful this is to others.
- Smile more.
- Express your gratitude to others. Say thank you. Be specific about what you're thanking them for and make clear how much you appreciate it.
- Show care and compassion towards others.
- Try to be objective and understand other people's points of view.
- If you have some free time, volunteer to give something back to your community. If you don't have much time, you could donate food to your local food bank or make a donation to a charity.
- Listen, really listen to others.
- Tell someone how they have inspired you, influenced you or made a positive difference to your life.
- Buy someone a small and thoughtful gift for no occasion, just a gift to celebrate them being who they are.
- Show more interest in people. Them as a whole. Not just in what they can do for you. Find out about their family relationships, what they've been up to, what they care about and what they're struggling with.
- Try to do one act of kindness per day. This can be something as small as holding the door open for someone in a rush.
- Give more hugs.

Being kinder to others and yourself can transform your life. If you practice kindness often, it becomes a way of life. You will think and act kindly automatically without any conscious effort.

Things to Look Forward To

We all need things to look forward to. Every culture in the world has annual celebratory events for the populous to look forward to. Everyone has individual things that they look forward to.

These may include:

- Going to music gigs, comedy gigs or theatre performances.
- Holidays, weekend or day trips.
- Time off work.
- Religious or Cultural celebrations, such as Christmas or New Year.
- Individual events, such as birthdays, weddings, anniversaries.
- Individual accomplishments, such as completing an academic courses, buying a property or completing a marathon.
- Visiting an attraction, such as a zoo, theme park, castle or other ancient site.
- Visiting a museum or art gallery.
- Visiting a place of historical significance.
- Episodes of a TV programme or seeing a particular film at the cinemas.
- Doing something special with family or friends.
- Changing weather, such as Spring bringing lighter, warmer days with plant growth.
- Getting a new piece of technology, such as a new smart phone, tablet or console.
- Attending a festival.
- The release of a book from an author you enjoy reading.

Having things to look forward to can be motivating, make us more enthusiastic about the future and prevent the feeling of being stuck in an unpleasant rut.

Write a list of things you've got to look forward to. Not much on it? Consider organising some things to look forward to. Try to spread the events out over the course of a year, so that you've always got at least one thing to look forward to.

Redefining Mental Health

Social media is like a hive mind. Got a question? Want an opinion? Ask social media. Whilst researching for the cover of this book, I asked on social media: **What images come to your mind when you think 'mental health'?**

Here are some of the comments:

"A black cloud."

"Darkness."

"Despair."

"Darkness, lonely and sad. Xx"

"Fear."

"I visualise a street looking from the bottom up. Gloomy and dull skies, wet pavements."

"Four walls with the curtains shut and daylight trying to seep through and an unhoovered carpet."

"A house with shutters slowly coming down and being boarded up. All light being extinguished and falling into total decay."

"Surrounded by people but still feeling alone. X"

"[The] image would be sat in space watching life going on and the earth turning but not feeling part of it anymore. Feeling alone and unwanted. A burden."

"Sadness not knowing what to do."

"Empty maps/squiggles."

"Think[ing that] you're going mad."

"Someone trapped in their mind."

"Anxiety always feel like I'm in a very small lift at braking point, feeling like I need to get out now *but I can't until I reach the next level."*

"A whirlpool of anxiety rotating in my solar plexus that is so strong it feels like it is physically there!"

"Absolute despair for the families. I'm speaking from experience. I have total sympathy for anybody who suffers with this terrible illness, but the first thing that comes to my mind is family despair and a feeling of complete hopelessness."

"Courage. Support. Fear. Xxx"

"But you don't *look sick."*

I was surprised by the responses. What struck me, is that that the responses were descriptions of mental illness *symptoms*, even though I'd asked about *mental health*.

We need to redefine the imagery of mental health. So if everyone associates it with a dark rainy cloud above someone, then what that someone needs is an umbrella. The darkness and deep shades of grey in the imagery, lightened up by the umbrella being brightly coloured.

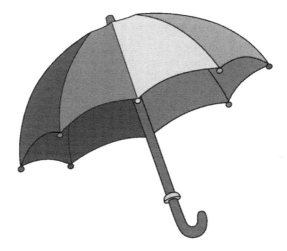

This is why the cover of this book has a brightly coloured umbrella on it, to change the imagery and associations. I've also made the umbrella deliberately bigger than the dark cloud on the cover, because there is more to someone than their mental illness.

While thinking about this umbrella imagery, I thought about what people need to be mentally and emotionally healthy and happy. I came up with 7 essentials:

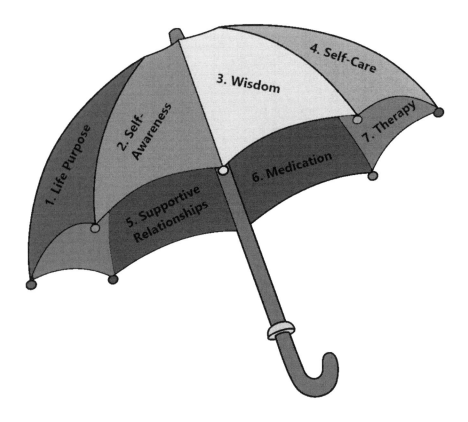

1. Life Purpose

Everyone needs at least one life purpose. A life purpose is something that you want to achieve over the course of your life.

People often describe it as *the reason you get up in the morning.* It's in your thoughts even when you are busy, what brings a feeling of happiness in your heart and what motivates much of your behaviour.

Here are some examples of life purposes:

- A cause - such as human rights or battling cancer. People usually find these causes through life experiences.
- Being kind to yourself and others.
- Caring for others - whether this be family members, friends, lovers or strangers.
- Community - we are social animals and have a deep need for community. These days you may be part of many communities, not just the community in the geographical area in which we live. A life purpose might be changing your community for the better or contributing to maintaining the community.
- Creativity - writing (books, poems, etc.), making music, making works of art (painting, sculptures, etc.), theatre (acting, developing shows, etc.), photography, films (acting, directing, etc.), basically making anything. It may be a specific piece of work you feel you were put on this earth to create or it may be a wide range of projects.
- Happiness - to experience happiness and joy as often as possible.
- Living your life being true to your values.
- Loving relationships - having connected, good and meaningful relationships with family members, friends and lovers.
- Making a positive difference to people's lives. This helps make the world a better place.
- Reproduction & Rearing - having children, grandchildren and great-grandchildren and raising them.
- Respect for nature and the environment.
- Striving for balance in all areas of your life.

- To accept and love yourself.
- To achieve your dreams.
- To be present in the moment.
- To be the best possible version of yourself.
- To have new experiences and get out of your comfort zone.
- To learn.
- To reach your potential.
- Travel - to explore the world.

My life purposes are to make a positive difference to people's lives, to care for others, creativity and happiness.

A life purpose isn't something that you're born with and that is your destiny to fulfil. People choose their life purpose, either consciously or unconsciously.

To help you identify your life purpose, answer the following questions and complete the sentences:

- What's the most important thing in my life?
- What about you are you most proud of?
- What always motivates you?
- If I died tomorrow, I would want people to remember me for...
- If you had to do one thing all day everyday for the rest of your life, what would it be?
- I'm most passionate about...
- My core values are...
- I would be happy if...
- I love anything to do with...
- I lose track of time when I'm thinking about or doing...

The ramifications of lacking a life purpose can be devastating. A lack of life purpose can contribute towards people struggling with addictions and mental illnesses.

2. Self-Awareness

There's a lot to being self-aware. But it starts with checking in with yourself. How do you feel physically? What are your thoughts? What are you feeling?

3. Wisdom

Wisdom is taking learning from knowledge and life experiences. Wisdom is what this book is all about. I hope that the contents of this book have given you greater wisdom around mental health and illness.

4. Self-care

Looking after your own mental health is really important. Hopefully having read this book you have more techniques and tips for self-care.

5. Supportive Relationships

All a child needs is one adult that loves and cares about them. It doesn't have to be their mum or their dad, they don't even biologically related. But adults are completely different.

As an adult, expecting one person to meet all your needs and wants is not only unrealistic, but a recipe for disaster. We need a wide range of supportive relationships to be healthy and happy.

6. Medication

As we get older our bodies need help to maintain normal functioning and deal with illness. One of the most common and scientifically-based treatments we use are medications.

Medications may be for our physical or mental health. If a qualified and experienced Doctor recommends a short course of medication or long-term medication to keep you in good health, then you should take it.

7. Therapy

Therapy can be an equally useful and effective treatment. This may be occupational, physio or talking therapies.

If you are offered therapy, take it and do the physical or mental exercises recommended.

If you have all these parts of your life sorted, you will be healthy and happy. If you find yourself feeling that you have all these parts sorted, but you are still unhealthy or unhappy, then you've overlooked something.

I hope that this book has been entertaining, informative and useful. I also hope that this book does what it is intended to do: make a positive difference to people's lives.

Acknowledgements

Acknowledgements

My mum has instilled me with confidence, fought battles to get the help and support I needed and loves me unconditionally. My mum is a constant inspiration to me. Mum, sometimes I see ways of thinking and behaviour in myself that are similar to yours. I couldn't emulate a better person. I love you now and always. Thank you for everything.

Papa you are a wonderful listener and brilliant at putting yourself in other people's shoes. I feel accepted and loved by you. Even when I was in hospital, at my worst, you not only visited me repeatedly, but showed me care, kindness and consideration. I will never be able to thank you enough, but thank you anyway. I am so happy that mum and you got together. You both deserve nothing but happiness.

My brother Neil is the most emotionally resilient person I know. Not only that, but he is one of the best examples of someone growing as a person I have witnessed. Thank you, brother, for the hugs, for listening, for advising, for the love and for the laughs. I smile every time I imagine you standing in that bin with a smile of pure joy on your face.

My soon to be sister-in-law Rhianne is confident, down to earth and radiates emotional warmth. Rhianne I loved you from the moment I met you. I absolutely adore you and love that you are joining our family. Neil: You are a very lucky man, never forget it.

Shaun, my long-lost brother. I think you were in my heart before we even met. I am so grateful for the chance encounter on the train between you and my mum. I am so pleased that you and Gill will be adding to our family.

Kelly, my annual vanilla candle supplier. Thank you for your unwavering support and countless brews.

Alex, my baby brother. You passed away far *too* soon and I miss you every day. Our relationship was incredibly special and I will always love you.

To the Watts Family - thank you all for adopting me, being there and including me in all aspects of your lives. Colin you are the father that I wish I'd had. Jenny you are my delight and confidant.

On to my dear friends. Sye you inspire me with your courage. Your encouragement and the way you live your life gives me much of my self-belief. Your illustration, radio voice, improvised comedy and acting skills are awesome. I'm so pleased that these aspects of you have been able to flourish.

Steve your determination and logical thinking are two of the many things I admire about you. You have gone above and beyond when it comes to supporting me, especially when I was in hospital. I thank you for your support and love that is without bounds. You are my tech support and without you I'd likely still be communicating with plastic cups and string. You've got a number of stories within you, I can't wait until they are shared with the world.

Jayne I felt an instant connection when we met, like we'd known each other forever. That connection is as strong as ever and unbreakable. You have such a deep well of kindness, compassion and empathy within you, I find it amazing and inspiring. I thank you for listening, for inspiring me and for being part of my life. I feel so lucky to have a friend like you.

Kay everyone should have a friend like you. Caring, warm and always there. We met because of geography, but bonded because of being kindred spirits. Thank you for sharing your unique perspective on life, for reminding me what's important in life and your kindness that you share with the world.

Simon, we are so alike in so many ways. Yet you are so much more. Wise, intelligent, empathic, funny and more earthy than I will ever be. It's great that I can turn up, anytime day or night and make myself at home in your home. I love our adventures and look forward to many more together. You have so many wonderful friends because of the warm, kind and engaging person that you are. Never stop being you.

Thank you to our National Health Service (NHS). It has saved my life three or four occasions, and the lives of my loved ones countless times. I am proud to live in a country where the access to healthcare that is of a high quality is not based on your bank balance; or on what level of cover an insurance company is willing to give you. Never let anyone tell you that we can't afford our NHS, *especially* not politicians.

Finally, I would like to thank the creators of Scrivener. I'm sure you have helped many authors to complete their manuscripts through your superb software. I remember seeing an acknowledgement to you, Literature & Latte, in one of Stephen Kings books. You must be so proud! It is the unique and simple organisation of my words that has helped to make this book, an idea I've had in various forms over years, a reality. Thank you.

Printed in Great Britain
by Amazon